FORENSIC MEDICINE –
A HANDBOOK FOR
PROFESSIONALS

FORENSIC MEDICINE – A HANDBOOK FOR PROFESSIONALS

Professor Alan A. Watson

GOWER
Aldershot. Brookfield USA. Hong Kong. Singapore.
Sydney

Published by
Gower Publishing Company Limited
Gower House
Croft Road
Aldershot
Hants GU11 3HR
England

Gower Publishing Company
Old Post Road
Brookfield
Vermont 05036
USA

British Library Cataloguing in Publication Data

Watson, Alan A., 1929–
    Forensic Medicine.
    1. Forensic medicine
    I. Title
    614'.1

ISBN 0 566 05513 9
Printed and bound in Great Britain at
The Camelot Press Ltd, Southampton

CONTENTS

List of Figures   x
Preface   xii

1 IDENTIFICATION OF AN INDIVIDUAL
   PERSON   1

   The Legal Responsibility   2
   Investigation by Police   3
   Identification to the Pathologist   3
   Procedure for Identification   4
   Identification by Personal Effects   5
   Identification by Facial Features   6
   Identification by Personal Defects and
      Peculiarities   7
   Identification from the Stature   12
   Estimation of Stature of Children   15
   Identification of the Sex   16
   The Determination of Age   25
   The Dating of Unearthed Human Bones   35
   Dental Identification   37
   Identification of Hair   38

v

	Fingerprints	39
	Contact or Occupation Data	40
	References	41

| 2 | POST MORTEM APPEARANCES | 42 |

	Lividity	43
	Rigidity	47
	Cooling of the Body	51
	Post Mortem Biochemistry	55
	Onset of Visible Decomposition	59
	Forensic Entomology	64
	Post Mortem Artefacts	67
	References	71

| 3 | THE POST MORTEM EXAMINATION | 72 |

	Request for a Post Mortem Examination	73
	The Medico-legal Autopsy	76
	Removal of Clothing from a Body	79
	The External Examination of the Body	82
	The Internal Examination of the Body	86
	The Refrigeration of Bodies	94
	The Effects of Embalming	94
	Exhumations	95

| 4 | DISPOSAL OF THE DEAD | 97 |

	Identification	97
	Cause of Death	98
	Registration of the Death	99
	The Death Certificate	99

The Informant 102
Disposal by Earth Burial 102
Disposal by Burial at Sea 103
Disposal for Medical Research 103
Disposal by Cremation 104
Disposal of Still-births 109
Disposal of Foetuses 110

5 SUDDEN AND UNEXPECTED
NATURAL DEATH 112

Cardiovascular System 113
Respiratory System 120
Central Nervous System 123
Gastrointestinal System 125
Other Systems 126
Sudden Death from Unknown Causes 127

6 WOUNDS AND INJURIES 128

The Distinction between a Wound and an
Injury 128
Some Fundamental Rules for Examining
Injuries 129
Some Fundamental Questions to be
Answered 131
Abrasions 134
Contusions (bruises) 139
Lacerations 146
Incised Wounds 150
Defence Injuries (Protective Injuries) 158
Penetrating Wounds 160
Summary 166

7 HEAD INJURIES   167

   The Fundamentals of a Head Injury   168
   Intracranial Haemorrhage   171
   Brain Swelling   179
   Concern for Head Injuries   179

8 ASPHYXIA   181

   Forms of Mechanical Asphyxia   182
   Forms of Toxic Asphyxia   198
   Forms of Environmental Asphyxia   202
   Forms of Medically Induced Asphyxia   204
   Forms of Pathological Asphyxia   204

9 INJURIES FROM PHYSICAL AND
   THERMAL AGENTS AND OTHER
   SOURCES   206

   Hypothermia   206
   Hyperthermia   211
   Injury and Death from Burning   213
   Burns from Chemical Agents   219
   Electrical Injuries   220
   Starvation and Neglect   226
   Wilful Neglect of Children   228
   Injury Due to Explosions   230
   Reference   235

10 FIRE CASUALTIES   236

   The Hazards of a Fire   237
   The Medico-Legal Aspects of a Fire Death   239
   References   252

11 FIREARMS AND FIREARM INJURIES   253

A General Classification of Firearms   253
Consideration of the Injury   269

12 DEATH IN CHILDHOOD   271

The New-born Infant   271
Sudden Infant Death Syndrome   278
Non-accidental Injury in Childhood   280
References   284

13 SEXUAL OFFENCES   285

General Legal Considerations   285
Medical Examination   289
The Clinical Examination   293
External Examination   294
Examination of the Genitalia   296
Examination of the Suspected Assailant   300
Examination in Cases of Anal Intercourse   302

14 DROWNING   305

Post Mortem Examination   307

SUGGESTED FURTHER READING   312

INDEX   313

LIST OF FIGURES

1.1	Sex differences in the pelvis	19
1.2	Sex differences in the pelvis (right innominate)	20
1.3	(a) Male pelvis showing narrow sub-pubic angle	21
	(b) Female pelvis showing wide sub-pubic angle	21
1.4	Sex differences in the pelvis (sacrum)	24
1.5	Male skull	26
1.6	Female skull	27
1.7	Mathematical sexing of the femur	30
1.8	Dental charts	34
2.1	Sites of pallor, supine position	44
2.2	Body in flexion due to heat	50
6.1	Mechanism of abrasion	136
6.2	Pattern of bruising caused by a vehicle tyre	140
6.3	Pattern of bruising caused by a cylindrical object	142
6.4	Laceration by a blunt object	148
6.5	Laceration caused by kicking	151
6.6	(a) Suicidal cut-throat	156
	(b) Self-inflicted incised wounds of the wrist	156

6.7	Stab wound	161
7.1	Sagittal section of head and intracranial haemorrhages	172
10.1	Characteristic 'pugilistic' attitude caused by prolonged exposure to heat	242
10.2	Division of body according to the 'rule of nines'	243
11.1	A high-grade double-barrelled sporting gun open ready for loading	257
11.2	A revolver open ready for loading	264
11.3	An automatic pistol	265
11.4	Types of pistol and revolver cartridges	267
11.5	Examination of recovered cartridge cases and bullet	268

PREFACE

FORENSIC medicine, and forensic pathology in particular, have for too long been considered to be the prerogative of a certain group of doctors, set apart for the awesome task. In novels, films, and now on television, the forensic pathologist continues to be portrayed as the sole custodian of certain vital and highly important facts, such as the precise cause of death. But we are not now in the realms of fiction.

Many professional people, not trained in medicine or the law, are finding themselves becoming steadily drawn to the subject, with a need to know in more detail some of the basic facts and principles of forensic medicine. Often such workers are required to prepare their own professional reports which include details of what happened to the victim. They need to have more than a vague impression of the subject.

This book is an attempt to meet the general needs of the professional worker, who stands alongside the doctor or the lawyer. He or she may be a police officer, possibly a detective, a fire service officer, a member of the nursing service, a precognition officer in a law office, a justice of the peace, or a member of the several paramedical professions who practise today.

The contents of the book are based not only on my formal university lectures to medical, law and nursing students, but also on lectures given to the Scottish Police College in the Detective Training Course, over many years.

I have endeavoured to reduce the enormous field of forensic pathology to a manageable size by emphasizing broad, but practical principles. There are many subjects left untouched, such as forensic odontology, the investigation of vehicular and aircraft accidents, all aspects of forensic psychiatry and the vast complex field of forensic toxicology. These can all be found in the large standard textbooks, specially written for the medical, legal and scientific practitioners.

This is a handbook, which I hope will be seen as such. At all times the needs of the professional worker have been to the forefront. It is sincerely hoped that the modest book will enable such colleagues to adopt a professional and clearer approach to the vast field of forensic pathology. In addition, on a practical level, it is hoped that they may be able to feel that they can discuss, uninhibited, cases and problems with the specialists, either in the post mortem room, or outside it. If this book can achieve all these aims, then I have succeeded.

I must acknowledge with deep gratitude the enormous help afforded me by my wife, Jean, who not only wrestled with the word processor and typed the manuscript, but has supported me wholeheartedly throughout the venture.

My sincere thanks must also go to my daughter-in-law, Margaret, who so kindly and readily offered to produce the illustrations for me.

Lastly I must express my thanks to the publishers and their staff for their faith in me at the beginning of the task and for their continued support thereafter.

A.A.W.
Glasgow 1988

1 IDENTIFICATION OF AN INDIVIDUAL PERSON

IDENTIFICATION means the indisputable recognition of a particular person which is based on certain unique and individual characteristics known to other people. Such characteristics are often quite small and unobtrusive, but their existence enables that person to be distinguished from all others. The question of the identification of a person frequently arises in both criminal and civil legal matters. The most simple problem is making an identification of a person from a witness box to the satisfaction of the court; a more difficult problem is that of selecting a person at a police identification parade. The medical and scientific aspects of identification are required with regard to the identity of a dead person, but occasionally these skills are demanded in civil cases, such as the identification of the father in paternity actions, cases of prolonged amnesia, or more rarely in identifying unknown persons allegedly impersonating long-lost relatives, seeking an inheritance or title.

We shall confine ourselves from now on to the problems of identifying a deceased person, and this will range from the recently dead person to a few fragmentary human remains.

We can subdivide the subject into the following classes, with increasing problems for a positive identification to be made.

1 Recently dead person
2 Decomposing body
3 Disintegrating body
4 Skeletal remains
5 Fragmentary remains

In practice, it is common to find some overlap of these classes. In a recently dead person it is usually a relatively simple procedure based on facial recognition by friends or relatives, but where, for a number of reasons the task is likely to prove difficult, the onus then lies with the pathologist. He will be required as part of his examination of the dead body to furnish a detailed description of the deceased's physical characteristics.

THE LEGAL RESPONSIBILITY

It is the responsibility of the procurator-fiscal or coroner to ensure that the identity of all dead persons discovered in their respective jurisdictions be established as far as it is humanly possible. This legal requirement is met by adopting a simple but formal procedure, namely of having some person look at the dead person and name the deceased before any post mortem examination is carried out. This formal act is important in eliminating any possible error or doubt, because it is worth remembering that, on occasions, administrative errors involving the identity of the body do occur by those responsible for handling the corpse, such as undertakers or mortuary attendants. Formal identification is the only safe way to unravel any confusion.

INVESTIGATION BY POLICE

WHEN an unknown corpse is discovered it falls to the police to make the first attempts at identification by discovering whether or not there are any personal objects in the clothing or about the body. The finding of personal papers, documents, identifiable jewellery or other items may supply the necessary information. It is surprising how frequently identification is established on information given by personal property; it then becomes a matter of police routine to notify relatives or friends of the deceased who, in turn, are requested to carry out formal identification. If the identification can be made without hesitation to the satisfaction of the police, this is accepted as conclusive and the details of the deceased are duly entered on the records.

IDENTIFICATION TO THE PATHOLOGIST

BEFORE an autopsy can be carried out, the body should be formally identified to the pathologist. It is most unsatisfactory for him to rely on the word of the mortuary attendant, ambulanceman or some other person who only had temporary access to the body. They may have good intentions but they may have been misinformed.

Identification can be made to the doctor in one of

3

two ways:

1   In Scotland it is customary for the witnesses who previously identified the body to the police, to re-identify to the pathologist before the autopsy.

2   Elsewhere the procedure usually adopted is: once the police have had a formal identification made to them they in turn will identify the body to the pathologist.

PROCEDURE FOR IDENTIFICATION

THE formal viewing of the body by relatives should be undertaken in an unhurried manner in a good light to obviate as far as possible mistaken identity, but it must be pointed out that many grief-stricken relatives find the formal occasion both distasteful and distressing. They are often too readily satisfied after only the sightest glance at the body. Such rapidity is obviously fraught with error, especially if, in the absence of a suitably designed viewing room, relatives are asked to identify the body on the mortuary table. It is not rare to find a witness who either cannot identify a close relative or makes a wrong identification. Be always sensitive to the feelings of the identifying witnesses.

To improve on the traditional method of relatives approaching the body, the Strathclyde Police have installed in the Glasgow City Mortuary a closed circuit television network. It has proved beneficial to all concerned and has been much appreciated by relatives. A two-dimensional view of the face in black and white removes some of the individuality of the deceased without losing the means of identification. It also has the unique advantage of enabling distressing face wounds or early signs of decomposition to be partially eliminated by a suitable arrangement of the head under the camera or by slight adjustments to the lighting controls. A recommended method of identification is to obtain the services, whenever possible, of persons who are not too closely related to the deceased, and are therefore unlikely to be too distressed by the appearance of the body.

IDENTIFICATION BY PERSONAL EFFECTS

MENTION has been made of the fact that personal effects such as the contents of a pocket may lead to a presumptive identity, which is subsequently confirmed by a visual examination of the deceased, but there are occasions when this latter examination is just not feasible. Victims of fires, explosions, accidents or extreme violence may have suffered such facial destruction or distortion that any hope of direct identification is out of the question. Identification of the clothing of the deceased, or of some unusual personal article may be the only way by which the owner will be known. Indubitably, there is considerable room for uncertainty and error, but frequently a parent will recognize various articles of a child's clothing, or a spouse will positively identify the rings of the deceased. Such methods should not go untried in difficult cases. Certain small articles, for example initialled handkerchiefs, are easily transferable between the various members of a family and therefore are unreliable for identification purposes. Whilst this form of identification is of only minor medical significance, it can be of considerable value to the police; in fact after visual identification of the body, this is the next most frequently used method. In a report by the Allied War Crimes Commission, which investigated many uncovered war graves in occupied Europe, it was stated that more than 60 per cent of victims were identified by items of clothing, many years after the bodies were buried.

IDENTIFICATION BY FACIAL FEATURES

RECOGNITION of the facial features is the method by which most bodies are identified. However, even in a recently deceased person, difficulties may be met, especially when the witnesses state that it has been a long time since they last saw the person alive. Frequently witnesses express considerable doubt and hesitation because the face in death differs so markedly from what they remember in life, even over a matter of a few days. The facial outlines are frequently altered by the mode of dying, by wasting diseases such as malignancy, following violence or by early post mortem decomposition. When a face is covered by blood, dirt or vomit, no identification should ever be made until after the face and head have been cleaned and made presentable, but before doing so, check that all the police photographic evidence has been satisfactorily recorded.

Despite these limitations, certain features of the face and head should be recorded as they may prove of value at a later stage. The state of the eyes and their colour should be recorded, together with any abnormalities such as a false eye, cataracts or other deformities.

The nature of the head and face hair should be described, paying attention to quantity, distribution, the texture, length, colour and any distinctive hair-styling. The facial hair should be noted with reference to whether the face is clean shaven or otherwise.

IDENTIFICATION BY PERSONAL DEFECTS AND PECULIARITIES

ON occasions, it has been found useful to consider the various personal defects seen on a body. In fact, the more pronounced and more uncommon the defect, the greater is its value. Such defects and peculiarities may best be considered under the following headings:

Bone defects

Old amputations, malunited fractures and deformities of the skeletal and muscular system, either from disease or from injury should be carefully recorded. The presence of old rickets with bowing of the legs, hunched or twisted backs, described kyphoscoliosis, unusual surgical operations and muscular atrophies, have all been used to establish a positive identification when more orthodox methods have proved impossible. The use of radiology, better known for its use in the detection of fractures in suspected crimes as well as in assessing the bone age of infants and children, can also be of value in comparing post mortem radiographs with those taken in life.

Skin defects

Unusual features on the skin must always be de-

7

scribed. Those of significance include the smaller abnormalities such as birthmarks, warts, pigmented moles and tumours as well as chronic skin diseases such as psoriasis, ichthyosis or even acne, for the reason that if they occur on the face or other exposed parts of the body, they would be readily noticed by relatives or friends.

Tattoo marks

These form a special class which on occasions have quickly established the identification, particularly when names or initials have been incorporated into the designs. The marks are produced by a hypodermic injection of a range of dyes which contain both stable and unstable pigments. The permanent stable dyes include carbon, India ink, Prussian blue and vermilion, whilst the less permanent pigments include cinnabar, cochineal, aniline dyes and ordinary inks. Most marks are to be found on the arms, but virtually the whole body surface has been used on rare occasions. The pictorial repertoire is relatively limited and predictable, showing service life, national, religious or family pride but sometimes most bizarre and erotic designs are seen.

> *Example* The naked body of a young man was found on waste ground with an unrecognizable face following a fatal frenzied attack. On one arm he had a fine tattoo of the badge of a Highland Regiment, whilst on the other arm the tattoo was that of a Lowland Regiment.

Such an unusual combination quickly led to his identification.

Example A badly mutilated body was recovered from the railway track following an accident with a passing train. On one arm there was a tattoo bearing the legend 'The only girl I ever kissed, was another man's wife – my mother'.

His identify was soon established by this means. All marks fade with age and certain colours, notably yellow, may completely disappear in periods varying from 20 to 50 years. A number of methods have been tried to eliminate marks, but total erasure can only be assured after radical surgery with possible skin replacement. Note any such attempts at erasure. Tattoo designs are sometimes altered by superimposition, but the results are usually far from satisfactory.

A point to remember is that on unknown decomposing bodies, for example on bodies removed from water, tattoo marks can be made more obvious, and thus suitable for identification and photography, if the loose epidermis is first removed, the colours and design details being thereby rendered more obvious.

Scars

It is important, occasionally, to consider the scars on a body in connection with identification, especially if they are the result of old injuries or unusual operations. If the original wound was a simple incision then one would expect to find only a thin linear scar because it would have healed by primary intention, but if the healing had been slow or delayed by infection with the formation of granulation tissue, then a prominent scar will be formed. For the first month the scar will appear red or brown because of the large

9

number of blood vessels in it but after a few months or even as much as a year later, the scar becomes firm, white and glistening. Unfortunately, the changes in the scar which occur after healing are too variable to serve as criteria for estimating the age of the lesion.

Some scars are *characteristic of the type of injury* which produced them.

(a) *Surgical scars* After certain operations, such as on the thyroid, the kidneys or the appendix the scars retain certain characteristic sizes and directions which distinguish them from other operations. With some abdominal incisions, accompanying pairs of tiny pinpoint scars, indicating the sites of deep tension sutures, as well as drainage stab wound scars are clearly visible.

(b) *Scars following violence* Attempted suicidal cuts to the neck or the front of the wrist show depressed horizontal scars of various sizes, their nature being in keeping with self-infliction. The scars of bullet wounds are seen as circular or slightly irregular skin depressions. Stab wounds often leave slightly elliptical scars which may appear elevated because of keloid formation. Severe lacerations often heal with large depressed irregular scars which may have deep attachments to the underlying structures such as bone. In the case of burns with much tissue loss broad and wrinkled scars have a tendency to produce tissue distortion and possible limitation of joint movement. Corrosive chemicals produce a similar result.

(c) *Scars from self-injection* The hypodermic injection scars of drug dependents must not be overlooked. Mostly they are circular, thickened and pitted as the result of small abscesses caused by unsterile injections. They should be looked for over the major veins of the forearms, the antecubital fossae and the thighs. Rarely other veins are used. In some female drug users, where the increased subcutaneous fat masks the underlying veins, the injections are sometimes made directly into the subcutaneous tissues of the back, the buttocks and other areas usually covered by clothing. Often the choice of sites requires the use of an assistant. The method is known as 'skin-popping' and produces large punched-out ulcers which heal with circular depressed scars.

(d) *Scars from natural diseases*   Many skin diseases such as acne and chickenpox, the smallpox vaccination marks and some chronic dermatoses may all leave characteristic scars on the skin which should not be overlooked. Following pregnancy and other abdominal enlargements, multiple, vertical linear scars, usually white and glistening, are seen on the abdominal wall and the upper thighs. These are known, following pregnancy, as striae gravidarum and result from over-stretching of the abdominal wall with rupture of the elastic tissue.

   The following two examples underline the importance of scars:

   Example   In a recent air disaster the bodies of four victims were found in a state of mutilation and disintegration. Identification was established in two bodies by the presence of scars. One person was known to have had plastic surgery to the inner aspect of both forearms several years earlier whilst the second body was found to have a circular scar on the side of the neck. It was later learned

11

that he had had surgery in childhood for cervical lymphadenitis.

Example A middle-aged female was reported missing several months before the remains of a headless and limbless torso was washed ashore. The remains comprised the spine, ribs and the skin of the chest and abdomen. All the internal organs were missing. Two surgical scars over the lower abdomen and left loin enabled a presumptive identification of the missing female to be made because she was known to have had a hysterectomy and a nephrectomy several years previously.

IDENTIFICATION FROM THE STATURE

WHEREAS the overall height of a recently dead or a partly decomposed but still intact body can be obtained by direct measurement, when one is dealing with skeletal material estimates have to be resorted to after taking certain appropriate bone measurements. It is obvious that the value of direct body measurements for identification purposes depends entirely on the existence of a record of the deceased's height taken during life. In many cases recordings of height taken in life are markedly inaccurate. Often they have been little more than estimates; at other times, doubts have been cast as to whether the measurement was the true height or the height in shoes. There are a few occasions when the actual height in life has been recorded, the best example being the measurement made for the purposes of life insurance. The age at which the recording or estimate was made is very relevant, as height may lessen with advancing age due to atrophic changes in bones and intervertebral disc cartilages.

When a body has been found in such a state of decomposition that disarticulation has occurred, a *rough estimate* of the stature can be obtained after the bones have been placed in their natural anatomical positions. The same degree of accuracy cannot, of course, be obtained as with an intact body but by making an allowance of from two to four centimetres for the superficial soft tissues and joint cartilage the estimate can be made. However, as was soon discovered as a result of the reconstructions in the Christie case, this method of estimating stature is open to considerable error since it is impossible to assess the thickness of the different soft tissues.

The only reliable method of estimating stature is by applying mathematical formulae to the length of the long bones. Since 1888 when Rollet published the first formula, based on 100 French men and women from Lyons, a number of similar formulae have been evolved for different populations. No physical anthropologist is fully content with the statistics so far produced, for as Trotter and Gleser indicated it is likely that different formulae may be required for the same racial group in successive generations; as it is, the present formulae are based on estimates of earlier populations.

The series of formulae, which most archaeologists and anthropologists use and therefore are commendable to forensic pathologists, were devised by Trotter and Gleser and are set out in Table 1.1.

The long bones are measured for accuracy in a Hepburn osteometric board, with all the bones in the vertical position, except the femur and the tibia which are measured in the oblique position. An

TABLE 1.1

Formulae by Trotter and Gleser (1952, 1958) for estimation of maximum living stature (cm), in Whites and Negroes, arranged in order of preference according to standard errors of estimate.

MALES

White	Negro
1.31 (Fem + Fib) + 63.05 ± 3.63	1.20 (Fem + Fib) + 67.77 ± 3.63
1.26 (Fem + Tib) + 67.09 ± 3.74	1.15 (Fem + Tib) + 71.75 ± 3.68
2.60 Fib + 75.50 ± 3.86	2.10 Fem + 72.22 ± 3.91
2.32 Fem + 65.53 ± 3.94	2.19 Tib + 85.36 ± 3.96
2.42 Tib + 81.93 ± 4.00	2.34 Fib + 80.07 ± 4.02
1.82 (Hum + Rad) + 67.97 ± 4.31	1.66 (Hum + Rad) + 73.08 ± 4.18
1.78 (Hum + Ulna) + 66.98 ± 4.37	1.65 (Hum + Ulna) + 70.67 ± 4.23
2.89 Hum + 78.10 ± 4.57	2.88 Hum + 75.48 ± 4.23
3.79 Rad + 79.42 ± 4.66	3.32 Rad + 85.43 ± 4.57
3.76 Ulna + 75.55 ± 4.72	3.20 Ulna + 82.77 ± 4.74

FEMALES

White	Negro
0.68 Hum + 1.17 Fem + 1.15 Tib + 50.12 ± 3.51	0.44 Hum − 0.10 Rad + 1.46 Fem + 0.86 Tib + 56.33 ± 3.22
1.39 (Fem + Tib) + 53.20 ± 3.55	1.53 Fem + 0.96 Tib + 58.54 ± 3.23
2.93 Fib + 59.61 ± 3.57	2.28 Fem + 59.76 ± 3.41
2.90 Tib + 61.53 ± 3.66	1.08 Hum + 1.79 Tib + 62.80 ± 3.58
1.35 Hum + 1.95 Tib + 52.77 ± 3.67	2.45 Tib + 72.65 ± 3.70
2.47 Fem + 54.10 ± 3.72	2.49 Fib + 70.90 ± 3.80
4.74 Rad + 54.93 ± 4.24	3.08 Hum + 64.67 ± 4.25
4.27 Ulna + 57.76 ± 4.30	3.31 Ulna + 75.38 ± 4.83
3.36 Hum + 57.97 ± 4.45	2.75 Rad + 94.51 ± 5.05

estimation based on the leg bones is more accurate than one based on the arm bones, and naturally, the more long bones that are measured the more accurate will be the estimate of the stature.

In practical terms, the stature is estimated by inserting the measured bone length into the formula and completing the mathematics.

For example if the length of the given femur is 45.0cm the equation, using the table given, will read 2.32 × 45.0 ± 65.53 ± 3.94cm = 173.87cm to 165.99cm. The addition or subtraction of 3.94cm is known as the *standard error of estimate*, similar to the standard deviation. In practical terms and using the given example ± approximately 4cm has a likelihood of 0/67 of being correct (i.e. two out of three cases will be correct) but an estimate of ± 8cm, which is twice the standard error, will have a likelihood of 0.95 of being correct (i.e. 19 out of 20 cases will be correct). The standard error of estimate is larger for some bones than for others. Hence in the formulae by Trotter and Gleser the bones have been arranged in an order of preference: the stature should be calculated from the bone which has the smallest standard error, that is, the one least likely to deviate from the actual height.

ESTIMATION OF STATURE OF CHILDREN

ANY attempt to estimate the length of a child from measuring individual long bones is rendered almost meaningless, because as there are so many variables that can affect the length of a growing bone, any estimates can never be more than mere approximations. Nevertheless, despite their rarity it is worth having the length of any discovered children's long bones recorded, because apart from the fact that the identity of the child and therefore its height may later be established, knowledge of the long bones in children is still very much at the stage of research.

IDENTIFICATION OF THE SEX

THE sex of an individual can be determined without difficulty if the external genitalia and the breasts are well preserved. Occasionally extra care is required in the case of new-born infants with minor development anomalies. Should such a problem arise this can be resolved either with the help of a paediatrician or by histological examination of the internal genitalia.

Difficulty may arise when decomposition of a body is so far advanced that both the external and internal genitalia have disappeared, either from exposure to air or water, after burial in the ground, as the result of mutilation and dismemberment, or when only portions of a body are available for examination. The problem is made more difficult if fragments of the body or mutilated remains are present which are not particularly diagnostic.

The *general characteristics* which distinguish the two sexes, quite apart from the genitalia and breasts may be summarized as follows.

The male is generally of larger and heavier build, showing greater muscular development, with more body hair, especially on the trunk and with less subcutaneous fat. He is broader at the shoulders than at the hips in contrast to the female where the hips are most pronounced. In the female the waist is quite distinctive but ill-defined in the male. The female buttocks are full and rounded but in the male they are more muscular and thus contractile and appear flatter. The limbs of the female are more rounded and gently contoured being covered by fine hair: the wrists, ankles, fingers, toes and nails are more refined in outline. The male fingers and toes are frequently very rugged. The distribution of the pubic hair in the female is generally limited to the mons veneris, whereas in the male it may extend upwards from the pubis on to the abdominal wall as far as the umbilicus, outwards on the inner aspect of the thighs and backwards along the natal cleft. In general, the hair of the male head is usually shorter, thicker and more coarse than that of the female, but this becomes unreliable in older age. The larynx of the male is more prominently developed than that of the female.

In making these general observations one must not overlook the uncommon case of the effeminate male or a masculine female where such distinctions are often very subtle.

With decomposition of the body the task is made more difficult but it is useful to remember that the non-pregnant uterus and the prostate are relatively resistant to rapid putrefaction.

Intensely hard and especially calcified tissues, such as fibroids and some biliary calculi, frequently seen in females, are often found unchanged, long after all the surrounding tissues are virtually indescribable, and these have all, on occasions, assisted in a presumptive sex determination.

In the absence of the sexual organs and distinguishing soft tissues it then becomes necessary to base the sexual distinction on the *secondary sex characteristics shown by certain of the bones*. In general, the bones of the female are lighter with thinner shafts and relatively wider medullary spaces than those of the male, and the sites for the muscle attachments are not so clearly defined. The pelvis, sacrum, sternum and skull are the bones most frequently examined to establish skeletal sex. In addition, measurements of some of the long bones can be used as confirmatory evidence.

Pelvis

Because the female pelvis is constructed for the function of childbearing, it usually presents very distinctive features enabling several contrasts to be made with the male pelvis (see Figures 1.1 and 1.2).

The pelvis gives the most reliable information of all and it is probable that a 90 per cent to 95 per cent accuracy can be achieved. The characteristics may be grouped into those depending upon naked eye examination; and those on which measurements can be made. General appearances can be noted.

1   The male pelvis is *robust* with well-marked roughened muscular attachment sites.

2   The *cavity* of the male pelvis is deep, but in the female it is shallow and wider.

3   The *walls* are widely splayed in the female.

4   The *obturator foramen* appears rather oval in shape in the male but is more triangular in the female.

5   The *pre-auricular sulcus* is absent in the male but quite obvious and sometimes pronounced in the female.

6   The *body of the pubis* is approximately triangular in the male but in the female it is almost square.

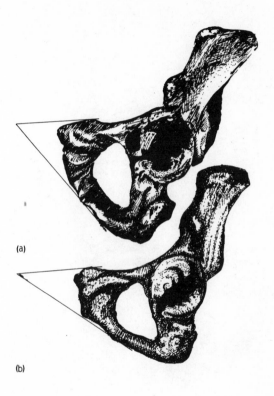

(a)

(b)

FIGURE 1.1   SEX DIFFERENCES IN THE
PELVIS, (a) MALE (b) FEMALE

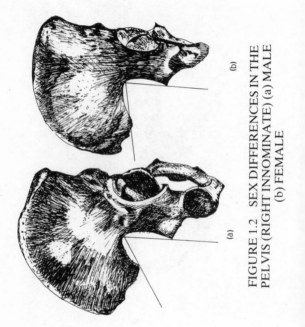

(a)

(b)

FIGURE 1.2   SEX DIFFERENCES IN THE
PELVIS (RIGHT INNOMINATE) (a) MALE
(b) FEMALE

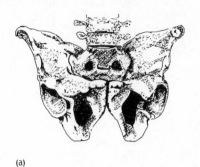

(a)

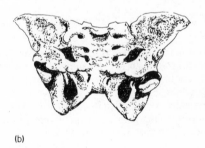

(b)

FIGURE 1.3(a)   MALE PELVIS SHOWING
NARROW SUB-PUBIC ANGLE (b) FEMALE
PELVIS SHOWING WIDE SUB-PUBIC ANGLE

7   The *pubic ramus* in the male is a continuation of the body of the pubis, in that it hardly changes its shape on the superior aspect, but in the female it has a pinched or 'waist-like' appearance.

8   The *great sciatic notch* is narrow and acutely angled in the male, open and large in the female appearing almost as a right angle and sometimes even as an obtuse angle.

The following *measurements* can be noted.

1   The *sub-pubic angle* of 90° or over (usually 100°) indicates the female sex. In the male the angle is about 65° to 75° (see Figure 1.3).

2   The angle of the *sciatic notch* is almost 90° and sometimes as much as 100° in the female, whereas in the male the angle is about 50° (see figure 1.2).

3   The *acetabulum* in the male averages 52mm in diameter but only 46mm in the female.

Sacrum

The sacrum of the male is long and narrow and may comprise more than five segments. The female sacrum by contrast is shorter and broader and as a rule has only five segments (see Figure 1.4). The difference in width is expressed by the sacral index. It consists of comparing the transverse diameter of the pelvic surface of the body of the first sacral vertebra with the transverse diameter of the base of the sacrum. The formula used is:

$$\frac{\text{Body width}}{\text{Basal width}} \times 100 = \text{Sacral index}$$

In general the index for males = 45.04 and for females 40.29.

In the female, the anterior surface is flattened in the upper part, followed in the lower part by an abrupt angulation forwards at the level of the fourth segment. In the male, the curvature is more evenly distributed over the whole length of the bone.

Sternum

In the male, the body of the sternum is at least twice as long as the manubrium, whilst in the female it is considerably shorter. This feature probably has an accuracy of 70 per cent. There is also the '149 Rule'. In Europeans, the combined midline length of the manubrium and sternum equals or exceeds 149 mm in males but is usually less in females. It has been estimated that this rule is accurate in at least 80 per cent of cases.

Skull

The sex of a subject can often be determined from certain characteristics of the skull (see Figures 1.5 and 1.6), but it is not easy if the skull is broken and fragmentary. Because of a certain degree of overlap of any one feature, the sum of all the characteristics should be considered with care. Nevertheless, the male skull may be distinguished from the female by reference to the following characteristics:

1   It is generally larger, rugged and less rounded. The female skull retains more of the adolescent form.

2   The supraorbital ridges are prominent, whereas in the female they are usually absent.

3   The mastoid processes are more pronounced.

23

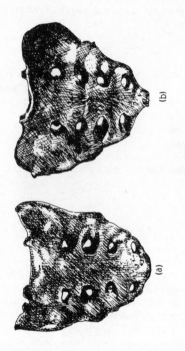

FIGURE 1.4   SEX DIFFERENCES IN THE
PELIVS (SACRUM) (a) MALE (b) FEMALE

4   The shape of the orbital cavities is rectangular, whereas in the female it is more circular.

5   The posterior root of the zygomatic process extends for some distance past the external auditory meatus as a well-defined ridge.

6   The mandible is more robust, with a broader ramus and a more developed coronoid process.

Long bones

The determination of sex from the long bones has been based for the most part on certain variations such as the size of the bones, the muscle-attachment areas and the weight and density of the bones. In general, these comments are applicable if a series of bones is being sexed; but if only one or two bones are available for examination, then it may be very difficult to draw any reliable conclusions.

A method for sexing a femur on a basis of certain measurements is shown in Table 1.2. See also Figure 1.7. The probability of attaining a correct result is greatly increased by the summation of these values.

THE DETERMINATION OF AGE

APART from its value in assisting in the identification of a dead person, the age of a person either living or dead may be required in several special medico-legal situations:

1   The maturity of the foetus, in relation to the crime of child destruction and the problem of viability.

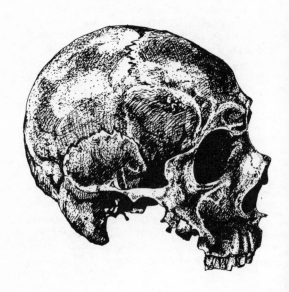

FIGURE 1.5   MALE SKULL

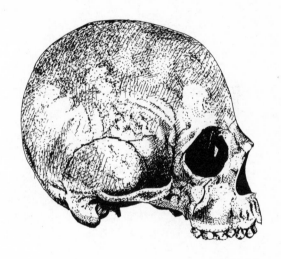

FIGURE 1.6   FEMALE SKULL

27

TABLE 1.2

MATHEMATICAL SEXING OF THE FEMUR

(Pearson and Bell, 1917–1919)

	Female (mm)	Female ? (mm)	Sex ? (mm)	Male ? (mm)	Male (mm)
Vertical diameter of head	41.5	41.5–43.5	43.5–44.5	44.5–45.5	45.5
Popliteal length	106	106–114.5	114.5–132	132–145	145
Bicondylar width	72	72–74	74–76	76–78	78
Trochanteric oblique length	390	390–405	405–430	430–450	450

2   In infants, in relation to child murder or infanticide.

3   In rape and other offences which depend on the age of consent.

4   The age of marriage and capacity for procreation.

5   In determining adulthood for various civil law matters e.g. eligibility to obtain work permits.

The skeleton and the teeth are the principal means whereby the age is estimated, but before discussing these factors, it is necessary to caution against being over-confident and giving ages which are too precise. It is far better to offer a relatively wide range of years, especially in the case of an adult, than give a totally misleading calculated age.

For the sake of simplicity and with increasing loss of accuracy, we shall consider three separate age groups. These are: the foetus and new-born child; from infancy up to 25 years; and adults over 25 years of age.

Development of foetus to new-born infant

End of 1st month –   length = 1.25cm (0.5in). Limb buds only are present

End of 2nd month –   length = 2.5cm (1in). Head with ears as well as hands formed. Ossification centres in clavicles and all shafts of long bones.

End of 3rd month –   length = 9–10cm (3.5–4in). Placenta formed. Nails appear. Ossification centre in ischium.

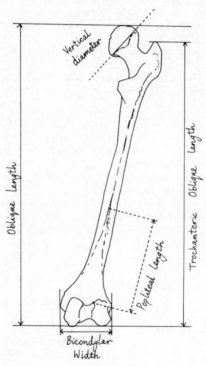

Right femur from behind

FIGURE 1.7 MATHEMATICAL SEXING OF THE FEMUR

End of 4th month – length 12.5–17.5cm (5–7in). Sex recognition. Ossification centre in superior ramus of pubis.

End of 5th month – length 15–25cm (6–10in). Ossification centre in calcanium. Growth of hair commences.

End of 6th month – length 22–30cm (9–12in). Umbilical cord situated just above pubis. Ossification centre in manubrium.

End of 7th month – length 32–37cm (13–15in). Nails do not yet reach ends of fingers. Foetus capable of life if born (legally viable). Ossification centre in talus and first segment of sternum.

End of 8th month – length 35–42cm (14–17in). Nails practically reach end of fingers, left testis in scrotum. Ossification centre at lower end of femur is just detectable. Centre in last segment of sternum.

End of 9th month – length 45–60cm (18–24in). Both testes in scrotum. Nails are fully formed. Ossification centre at lower end of femur is about 5mm in diameter and there may be a small centre seen at upper end of tibia.

A *rule-of-thumb calculation* for the foetal age from the end of the fifth month is obtained by dividing the length of the foetus in centimetres by 5. This will give the age in months. For example:

$$\text{foetal length} = 35\text{cm divided by } 5 = \text{end of 7th}$$
$$\text{month.}$$

The new-born infant

The main medico-legal concern is in deciding whether or not the infant was legally viable (born after 28th week of pregnancy) and if viable, whether the child was sufficiently mature to withstand the difficulties of delivery and a separate existence. Conclusions are based on the weight and length of the infant and the distribution of the skeletal ossification centres.

Thus at 28 weeks (legal viability) the vortex-heel measurement should be 35cm (14in) with a range of 32–37cm (13–15in) and ossification centres are visible in the talus and first segment of the sternum.

When centres are found not only in the talus but also in the calcaneum, the cuboid and the lower end of the femur then it can be stated with certainty that *the infant was mature at birth*.

During the first 36 hour the umbilical cord dries, and from 36 to 48 hours a clear ring of demarcation can be seen forming around the junction of the cord and the abdominal wall. The stump blackens and sloughs off at about seven days forming a well-healed scar in about 10 days.

Childhood to early adulthood

(i) *Dentition*   An estimation of age with reasonable

accuracy can be made for the period beginning at about six months up to about 21 years. Such accuracy is based on the respective times of eruption of the individual temporary and permanent teeth. The dental charts (Figure 1.8) indicate the approximate dates at which the different teeth appear.

(ii) *Ossification centres*   Brief mention has already been made of selective bones in which certain centres of ossification can be seen, thereby determining the approximate age of a foetus or a new-born child. From birth up to at least five years, other primary ossification centres can be found. These range from the head of the tibia at from one to four weeks, to the lower end of the ulna at five years. Their presence is seen relatively easily by radiology, but the interpretation of the results is best left to the radiologist.

(iii) *Fusion of epiphyses*   Up to the age of about 18 to 20, an estimate of the age may be given by the fusion of the epiphyses of the bones to their shafts. The times of fusion generally follow a definite order but there is considerable individual variation. The accuracy increases with the number of observations made. As with the ossification centres, the determination of fusion of epiphyses is best left to the radiologist to avoid misleading calculations.

Adults over 20 years

Beyond the age of 20, the ageing of an unknown body becomes increasingly more difficult, and it is doubtful whether one can get closer than within ten years when presented with skeletal remains alone. Former-

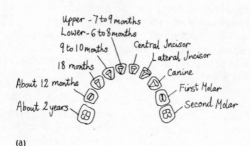

(a)

(b)

FIGURE 1.8 DENTAL CHARTS
(a) TEMPORARY OR DECIDUOUS TEETH
(b) PERMANENT TEETH

ly, standard textbooks placed much emphasis on timing of the closure of the sutures of the skull and even short tables were produced. New data made available from examinations of soldiers killed in Korea has shown that suture closure is so highly variable that it is of little use as a guide for determining age. It seems best, therefore, to disregard former teaching on skull sutures. Some successes have been reported using the rugged appearances of the faces of the pubic symphysis; and comparisons can be made with publicized tables but so far the work has been limited to males in the younger age groups.

Other changes occur as part of the natural ageing process. There is ossification of the costal cartilages and in the larynx, and probably the most obvious are the degenerative changes that occur to the cartilage lining of weight-bearing joints of the spine and legs. All these changes may occur between 40 and 70 years and whilst they herald old age, they by no means give precise information.

THE DATING OF UNEARTHED HUMAN BONES

WITH the continuing expansion in the national building programme and in road development, human skeletal remains are frequently unearthed. They are recovered in most unusual sites and at variable depths. Before becoming involved in an investigation it would be wise to consult a large-scale map of the area to see whether there are any sites likely to be of antiquarian or archaeological interest.

Bone material may be found in a number of geological areas. These include sands, clays, river gravels and peat bogs. The sites may include various burial earthworks, old buildings, battlefields, plague pits, old cemeteries, caves or underground shelters. Consultations with local historians, libraries, archaeologists and anthropologists may shed some light on the problem. The importance of attempting to estimate the age of any unearthed bones is that the police, Procurator Fiscal or Coroner will want to know whether the remains are recent enough to warrant undertaking further enquiries, or are of sole interest to the archaeologists. The dividing line is usually taken to be 75 years or even slightly higher. If the bones appear to be older than 75 years then they become of little legal interest, because if there is the possibility of a homicide, the chances are that the perpetrator of the crime is also dead.

The preservation of bones varies considerably not only from soil to soil but, because of minor soil differences, from one site to another in the same area. In permeable gravel soils, where the acidity is high, the bones are poorly preserved, in contrast to the anaerobic, water-logged, peaty conditions where the bones are stained dark brown and well preserved. In chalky and sandy soil, the bones may show a considerable degree of erosion usually at the joint surfaces and the bone substance is light and very fragile. Clay soil is unpredictable.

The presence of ligaments and cartilage suggest a recent death, usually less than a year, whilst periosteum is frequently seen on bones buried up to ten years or more. With bones over ten years, there is just a trace of the odour of decay but that depends on climatic factors. If strong, the odour is a reasonable indicator of a recent death.

There is a series of laboratory tests which can be

used and whilst each test on its own is of little practical value, when used in combination with others they do point to some very general conclusions. For example, the human precipitin reaction gives positive results for up to about five years after death whilst thin-layer chromatography and ultra-violet fluorescence may be used up to about 100 years after death. It must be concluded that realistically the dating of unearthed bones is not accurate, so that having regard to all the available evidence, one is led to make nothing more than an inspired and intelligent guess!

DENTAL IDENTIFICATION

AN examination of the teeth may prove to be of considerable value in the identification of the recent dead and of skeletal remains, because both the temporary and permanent dentition are almost indestructible by the normal processes of putrefraction and composition. Only an intense fire can destroy them. This fact makes dental inspection an important part of identification in mass disasters, domestic fires and other similar catastrophes.

Whenever possible the charting of the teeth, the description of any dental peculiarities and particulars of dental work, together with the taking of impressions, casts and dental X-rays should be performed by a competent dentist or preferably by a forensic odontologist.

After all the particular characteristics of the teeth and jaws have been duly recorded, the details may then be compared with the professional records of the deceased's dentist, if and when they are made available. But even accurate charting has a value only to the extent to which data are available for comparative study. It is exceptional for a dentist to establish an identity simply on a general circulation of dental data around dentists, for it would necessitate checking through very large numbers of records. Even the NHS dental records are retained for only a relatively short time before being destroyed.

The recovery and identification of dentures together with any existing teeth have been responsible for the identification of many people, especially in mass disasters such as aircraft crashes or shipping accidents. The marking of dentures by dental technicians and laboratories is not yet commonplace but where it has been done, it has proved to be most useful.

In recent years the evaluation of bite marks has played a decisive role in identification in a criminal context. Unfortunately because of the relative rarity of bite marks, few authorities have studied more than a mere handful of cases, and because of this all bite marks will be examined only by forensic odontologists. Although each mouth has its own special characteristics, the differences in the position and size of teeth are usually small and therefore it is necessary that impressions of the mouth and the bite mark be taken and moulds and casts prepared for comparison.

IDENTIFICATION OF HAIR

HAIR from an unknown person can be compared in the laboratory with a sample of known hair, and whilst it is not yet possible to state categorically that the two hairs under comparison originated from the same source, we are often in a position to say that the two samples of hair could not possibly have come from the same person.

Some common situations where hair studies are made include the finding of hairs on the front of a car or a train following an accident, to be able to link the vehicle with the victim. In cases of sexual offences, the demonstration of unusual hairs on clothing or on the pubic hair of an accused may help to lead to a conviction. In a recent mass air disaster, the identity of one person was confirmed by comparing hair from the mutilated head with samples of the suspected person's hair obtained from his comb and hairbrush at his home.

In sending hair to the laboratory it is advisable to pluck out hair by the roots rather than cutting off the distal two or three inches. The examination of the proximal portion of the hair is more reliable than the distal part. Head hair is remarkably resistant to decomposition. Whilst it may be found completely detached from the scalp in advancing decomposition, the individual hairs remain almost unchanged and therefore suitable for examination for a considerably long period.

FINGERPRINTS

THIS unique method of identification is performed only by the Identification Branch of the police. It is now an extremely sophisticated science, backed up by computerized data retrieval. From the point of view of the general reader it is worth remembering that apart from finger- and palmprints, impressions from the sole and the lips can be examined but it remains a less exact science. Even with decomposing bodies when the epidermis is being shed, the recording of fingerprints from the deeper skin layer is still of value, but often the results are difficult to read.

CONTACT OR OCCUPATION DATA

Recent and temporary

Contact traces of material with which the deceased worked before his death have, on occasions, been of corroborative rather than direct evidential value in the process of identification. Such traces have included paints, varnishes, different oils and greases and sawdust. Microscopical examination and toxicological analysis are required before any reliance can be placed on these substances.

Example The partially skeletalized body of a man was found in some woods. Before his disappearance he had worked in a sawmill on the other side of the woods. In his two ears were found traces of sawdust, which on botanical examination showed them to have come from a very soft wood, probably fir or pine. Whilst the woods contained a mixed population of trees, the sawmill had been used six months earlier on a batch of pine trees. Thus the man was linked with the mill and a presumptive identity was made.

Longstanding and permanent

Such features are of limited value, but occupational traits such as coalminers' dust disease in the lungs or some other pneumoconiosis, or the callosities found on the skin of the hands in association with certain trades and crafts may, like the occupation data above, play a corroborative role in identification.

REFERENCES

Pearson, K. and Bell, J.A. (1917–1919), *Draper's Company Research Memoirs*, Dept. of Allied Statistics, Cambridge University Press, Chaps. 1–4.

Trotter, M. and Gleser, G.C. (1952), *Am. J. Phys. Anthrop.*, Washington (N.S.) **10**, 463–514.

Trotter, M. and Gleser, G.C. (1958), *Am. J. Phys. Anthrop.*, Washington (N.S.) **16**, 79–123.

2 POST MORTEM APPEARANCES

VERY shortly after death, there begins a series of biological changes, the first steps in the process of decomposition which, because of their gradual onset, may be used to calculate the length of the post-mortem period. Expressed another way, these body changes help us to form an opinion as to the time of death. But it must be said straight away that these biological changes can vary quite considerably in otherwise similar bodies, to the extent that any result obtained for a specific body must be regarded as rather imprecise. Furthermore, a calculation made is only of value for a period of up to about two days. Beyond that time, the calculation becomes little more than guesswork and is best expressed as 'a rough estimation of the duration of the post mortem period.'

The three main changes which provide the most useful values, however, imprecise, and which should always be considered collectively before expressing an opinion, are:

1 *Lividity* (livor mortis, post mortem staining, hypostasis)

2 *Rigidity* (rigor mortis, muscular stiffening)
3 *Cooling of the body* (algor mortis)

Other less reliable methods include:

4 Alteration to the body fluid biochemistry
5 Onset of visible decomposition
6 Invasion by insects

LIVIDITY

THE term refers to the reddish purple discolouration in the skin of the dependent parts of the body, caused by the gravitational pooling of de-oxygenated blood within the small blood vessels. It will, of course, not be seen in those areas where firm contact is made between the body and the underlying surface or where the skin is bound by constrictive clothing. Consequently, when a body is discovered lying on its back, an examination of the back will show contrasting areas of white skin and of a red-purple colour (see Figure 2.1). The usual sites of pallor are the regions of the shoulder blades, the buttocks, the back of the calves, the elbows, the heels and the back of the head or even under clothing such as the straps of a brassiere. These are the areas of contact which support the body in the supine position.

When a body is discovered fully or partially clothed and some of the clothes have become rucked up at the back by folds and creases, new, additional foci of contact pressure are produced, thereby adding new patches of pallor in sites where one expects to see nothing but hypostasis. Alternatively these foci of pressure, by lessening the pressure in the areas adjacent to the foci, may allow additional unexpected

43

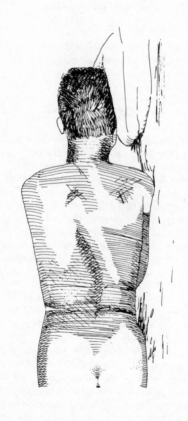

FIGURE 2.1   SITES OF PALLOR, SUPINE
POSITION

areas of hypostasis to appear. Thus when clothes become disarranged in a fight or in a struggle preceding death, they may produce irregular lividity patterns which may become quite important. (To distinguish hypostasis from bruising see Chapter 6.)

Slight variations in colour from the usual reddish purple hue are frequently seen and this is normal. Such variations depend on pre-existing anaemia, jaundice and respiratory or cardiac failure with associated cyanosis. There is however, one important colour variant which must not be overlooked because of its medico-legal importance and that is *bright pink verging on cherry red*. This colour change in the dependent skin suggests one of three possibilities:

1   Carbon monoxide poisoning
2   Cyanide poisoning
3   Hypothermia and exposure

In cases of poisoning by carbon monoxide or cyanide, the colour change results from chemical alteration, or enzymatic damage to the process of oxygen combining with haemoglobin and its subsequent release to the tissues. With regard to hypothermia, such as cases where there is rapid cooling after death brought about by thinly clothed bodies lying in a cold, wet environment, there is a poor release of oxygen to the tissues at the time of death. This results in much residual oxyhaemoglobin.

Lividity is normally clearly perceptible as purplish blotches within an hour of death and in some thin individuals the first changes appear in the lumbar region very shortly after death. The intensity of the purple colour and its distribution increase steadily for up to twelve hours when maximal intensity is attained. Up to this time, the fluid blood may be moved around, so that if the position of the body is changed, there will be fading of the colour from the former dependent areas and a reappearance in the new sites. This feature of altered lividity with body interference may be used, with caution, to assert that a body has been moved since death. A simple test for the displacement of lividity is to apply finger pressure on a purple area for a few seconds, when the colour can be made to blanch. After about twelve hours the discolouration begins to 'fix' in the vessels, due partly to coagulation of some of the blood, but also caused by hardening of the connective tissue fat around the blood vessels. The question as to whether or not the hypostatic blood can be moved is certainly not one that will help determine the time of death.

An associated phenomenon, known as 'Tardieu's spots', is sometimes seen in areas of intense lividity. The term was originally applied by Tardieu to sub-pleural petechial haemorrhages present in association with asphyxia but the term is now also used to describe multiple, sometimes confluent, small haemorrhages which are the result of agonal or post mortem rupture of engorged and distended capillaries. The subsequent leakage of blood is drawn close to the skin surface by gravity.

Hypostasis also occurs in the internal organs. One example is the intense congestion seen in the basal and posterior areas of the lungs, and care must be taken by the pathologist to avoid attributing this change to pulmonary congestion secondary to left ventricular failure, or to haemorrhagic pneumonia or some other natural disease. In the case of the heart, lividity appears in the myocardium of the postero-lateral walls of the left ventricle. To the unwary, this normal process, when exaggerated, may be mistaken for an early myocardial infarction, especially in the presence of severe coronary atherosclerosis.

RIGIDITY

THIS refers to the stiffening or hardening of the muscle after death with increasing muscular contraction and fixation of the joints. There is coagulative necrosis of the cytoplasm of the muscle cells, the onset of which depends on the pH of the muscle tissue and the gradual disappearance of adenosine triphosphate from the muscle. The lowering of the pH is dependent largely on the amount of glycogen reserve in the muscle and the rate of exhaustion of the oxygen available to the muscle. The rigidity increases with the acidity and may be detected in an early stage as early as 30 minutes after death, especially if, just before death, the deceased had been exercising vigorously or having convulsions.

The onset of rigidity, as determined by a limitation of joint movement, has been stated to begin in the muscles of the face and progress steadily downwards. What does occur is, first, fixation of those joints which are surrounded by a small muscle mass, followed in turn by those joints surrounded by increasingly larger muscle masses. Therefore, rigidity will first be seen in the muscles of the face, the lower jaw, the fingers and toes, followed by the elbows, knees, wrists and ankles, leaving the hips, shoulders and back to a later time.

Muscular rigidity is discernible in the medium sized muscle masses, such as the arms, two to three hours after death and progresses steadily to reach a maximum over the entire body somewhere between six and twelve hours after death. The wide time-scale noted depends very much on one's own ability, first, to assess the degree of rigidity reached and in particular where any change has occurred since the last assessment; second, to physically lift and manipulate the limbs of a heavy, muscularly built man.

Some other factors that need to be considered include the rapidity of body cooling: the faster the rate, the slower the onset of rigidity; the degree of muscular development and the state of muscular activity just before death. In the case of a new-born baby, with very little muscular development, the onset of rigidity is very rapid and its duration is relatively short.

The disappearance of rigidity is probably more variable than its onset. It begins to disappear in as little as 18 to 24 hours after death, especially if the body has lain in a hot environment, accelerating the rate of decomposition, or it may remain virtually unaltered for up to five or even six days if left lying in cold conditions. Whilst environmental temperature is clearly of importance, so also is it important to recognize that little reliance can be placed on rigidity alone as a means of estimating the time of death.

Once rigidity has reached its maximal intensity and then been forcibly 'broken down', by manipulation of the joints, or rough handling of the limbs, it cannot recur. The muscles proceed to early decomposition. This fact may be of some significance to criminal investigations by suggesting that because of the combined presence and absence of rigidity in an irregular fashion, the body may have been manhandled after death.

It is often forgotten that rigidity also affects the musculature of the internal organs, in particular the heart. If a post mortem dissection is carried out between six and twelve hours after death, the myocardium is firmly contracted. This could make an evaluation of the heart valves somewhat difficult, especially if the mitral valve is said to be clinically diseased. Rigidity may also give a false impression as to whether the thickness of the ventricular wall is really sufficiently increased to justify the pathologist calling it hypertrophied.

Other organs include the urinary bladder and the large intestine, but rarely does the rigidity interfere with the examination of these organs.

There are three special forms of rigidity.

Effects of freezing

When a person dies in freezing conditions, it is common for the body to show total rigidity due simply to the process of freezing which has taken place *before* the onset of true rigor mortis. After such a body is thawed out, the body will then show the initial flaccidity which occurs immediately after somatic death. Rigor mortis will then begin in the normal way reaching its maximum fairly rapidly and passing off equally rapidly.

Effects of excess heat

Bodies recovered from fires, apart from very severe charring of the superficial tissues, often show very marked flexion contractures of the muscles and limbs (see Figure 2.2). The imbalance between the flexor and extensor muscles causes the body to adopt the 'pugilistic' attitude. When seen for the first time one

49

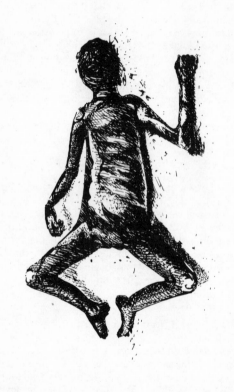

FIGURE 2.2 BODY IN FLEXION DUE TO HEAT

may think that the victim was in a 'fight or flight' situation, especially when compounded by skin splitting on the limbs which greatly resembles incised wounds. They are mere post mortem artefacts caused by heat coagulation with gross contracture of the major muscle masses (see Chapter 10 and Figure 10.1).

Cadaveric spasm

This is a rare form of excessive rigidity produced in only a limited part of the body at the moment of death, when the victim has been under extreme physical, mental or emotional stress. Soldiers killed on the battlefield have been found still tightly holding some piece of equipment, e.g. rifle, or a hand grenade. Also reported are cases of suicides still holding the weapon with which they have killed themselves. The significance of this finding is that it is presumed that the wounds caused by the grasped weapon must have been self-inflicted. Whilst the biochemistry involved in the muscles of the limb or limbs affected is still far from clear, the degree of rigidity appears to be maximal from the onset and passes off more slowly than the normal rigidity noted elsewhere.

COOLING OF THE BODY

THE loss of heat from a body is one of the earliest observations to be made after death. For many years pathologists have attempted to record the changing temperature and from the graphical curve obtained they have proceeded to estimate the time of death, at least within the first twelve hours.

Marshall and Hoare, in an extended series of cases, established that the cooling curve, as measured rectally, has a slightly sigmoid shape with an initial plateau followed by a straight portion and then ending with a curved gradient.

To record body cooling differences, a chemical thermometer is usually used. Under research conditions an electrical recording device using microwave thermographic detectors or other similar probes linked to a computer and a print-out machine have been used. A clinical thermometer is completely useless. The measuring device must be inserted into the rectum to a distance of at least four inches in order to record the inner 'core' temperature. The outer core, or outer layers, of the body, which account for approximately 50 per cent of the body mass, have a significantly lower temperature and can be more easily influenced by alterations in the conditions of the environment. If possible, several readings should be taken from the same site, to produce a simple cooling curve. Sophisticated recording devices, although of value in research, at the moment have little application to the clinical or the forensic pathologist called to see the body at the locus. We await technical advances. The body cools by radiation, conduction and convection, and because of its complex nature, the rate of cooling cannot be expressed as a simple exponential curve. Marshall and Hoare have produced a formula, which is virtually unworkable, from a series of exponential terms, but they have suggested the following points:

1   There must be established after death a regular flow of heat from the inner core, through the more resistant outer core, to the surface. Until this has taken place, and it generally requires between one

and three hours, there is relatively little internal cooling.

2   During the next six to nine hours, the heat flow is maintained at a steady rate so that the internal cooling is rapid.

3   After six to nine hours, the skin temperature approaches the environmental temperature and only then does the rate of body cooling follow a simple exponential curve.

4   In practice the curves calculated by Brown and Marshall and published in standard textbooks of forensic medicine should be consulted.

5   A rough rule, but quite useful, described by Knight assumes the temperature of the body to be 37°C and the difference between this temperature and the rectal temperature is the degree of cooling. This degree of cooling is then multiplied by 1, 1.25, 1.50, 1.75 or 2 according to an ambient air temperature of 0°, 5°, 10°, 15° or 20°C respectively. The resultant figure is the time in hours elapsed since death.

6   An even simpler rule is to accept an average fall in temperature of 1°C per hour. The resultant 'time of death' can be altered by assessing the conditions at the place where the body was found.

The following factors should not be overlooked because they will influence the rate of cooling.

Obese body

A body possessing a large amount of deep and subcutaneous fat will cool more slowly than a lean body, because the ratio of body mass (weight) to surface area is altered. The more spherical and less cylindrical the body, the slower the rate of cooling. There is simply more bulk to cool.

It is sometimes said that the reason for the slowing of the rate of cooling is that fat is a poor conductor of heat. This is just not true; fat cools at the same rate as non-fatty tissue, other things being equal. The confusion may arise because of trying to equate the presence of fat in the living with that of the dead. In the living, because subcutaneous fatty tissue is less vascular than subcutaneous muscle, the rate of heat loss at the skin surface is slower. Hence the need for fat or fat substitutes in cross-channel swimmers, to help reduce the rate of heat loss. After death, however, vascularity plays no further part, and fat and muscle cool at the same rate.

Therefore, in an obese body we are concerning ourselves with the simple physical properties of mass versus surface area.

Thin body

An emaciated body or one with an abnormal physical build has a larger surface area relative to its mass, thereby increasing the rate of heat loss.

Original body temperature

Occasionally persons die with markedly high temperatures. In some cases of heat stroke, the post mortem rectal temperature has been observed to rise for over half an hour after death up to 110°F (44°C) before cooling began. Similarly in hypothermia, abnormal initial readings may disturb the estimation considerably, the body temperature *at death* being considerably lower than normal.

Environmental temperature

The temperature of the immediate environment of the body will greatly affect the rate of cooling. The presence of insulating material, such as clothing, bedding, electric blankets, hot room, on the one hand, and nudity, dampness, soil, wind, rain on the other hand will slow down and accelerate cooling respectively.

> *Example*   A woman died in a sauna from natural disease. The temperature of the sauna was 140°F. When discovered nearly four hours later the body was hot to the touch and was showing decomposition changes, suggesting that death had occurred at least four days previously.

In summary, it should be abundantly clear that the results obtained from temperature readings, environmental and physical factors and the resultant cooling graph can only achieve a very general opinion as to the time of death. It requires the taking of body temperatures on many bodies in order to begin to appreciate the uncertainties in the post mortem body temperature. Confidence can only come with practice and repeated readings taken at the locus.

POST MORTEM BIOCHEMISTRY

BIOCHEMICAL analysis of blood, cerebrospinal fluid and vitreous humour may be of medico-legal significance in several ways:

1   Biochemical studies may establish a cause of death in the absence of any significant morbid anatomical or pathological abnormality.

2 Such studies may demonstrate a cause of death, or at least show the ante mortem state, in those cases where an autopsy cannot or may not be performed.

3 They may help to link up clinical findings with subsequent pathological findings.

4 Post mortem chemistry may combine with other methods in establishing the time of death.

An important review article by Coe (1974) presented all the main aspects of post mortem chemistry and it has remained a compendium of the available date. The summary of all the findings contains the comment that perhaps the only chemical analysis having more than the slightest value in determining the post mortem interval is that of vitreous humour potassium levels. One other test worthy of a mention is the combined results of amino-nitrogen, non-protein nitrogen, creatine and ammonia in both plasma and cerebrospinal fluid.

If the time of death aspect of post mortem chemistry is disregarded, then some chemical studies may still have a role in medico-legal cases.

Alcohol levels in vitreous humour

These follow very closely the serum values and may be used when there is a question of possible contamination of blood samples, or when the body has been so severely mutilated that blood is impossible to obtain in an unsoiled condition. The use of vitreous humour is very useful in embalmed bodies, in which alcohol plays an important role, and also where the body has been rendered useless by decomposition.

Study of hormone levels

Post mortem cortisol levels may help to exclude
Addison's disease in the presence of hypoplastic
adrenal glands. Thyroid function tests on post mortem serum have been of value in severe chronic thyr-
oiditis. But insulin levels have been shown to be too
variable to have any practical value.

Post mortem enzyme determination

Most enzyme levels rise after death: the phosphatases, amylase, transaminases and in particular lactic
dehydrogenase. The latter has been found to have a
roughly linear increase in concentration against time
during the first 60 hours after death. It has been suggested that this might be helpful in estimating the
post mortem interval.

Post mortem blood cholinesterases remain stable
for prolonged periods and these could have significance in cases of toxic hepatitis where in life there is
a marked drop in the enzyme level.

Lipid substance

Cholesterol and other serum lipids have been shown
to be stable in post mortem blood with little loss due
to autolysis, and some correlations between the
levels of post mortem lipid substances and the discovery of unsuspected coronary artery disease have been
made.

Serum proteins

By immuno–electrophoresis it has been shown that the post mortem serum fractions accurately reflect the state of the proteins in life. Such studies have been used to demonstrate hypogammaglobulinaemia and specific electrophoretic findings of myeloma.

Electrolytic studies on vitreous humour

Studies on vitreous humour reflect fairly closely electrolytic variations in ante mortem blood, and the humoral levels remain constant for a prolonged post mortem time. This has particular reference to sodium and chloride levels. Coe demonstrated hypernatraemia and hyperchloraemia in cases of neglect in both children and adults. In the presence of pyloric obstruction with prolonged vomiting he used vitreous humour to show depressed sodium and chloride levels. Other electrolytes have been studied such as phosphorus, calcium and magnesium but the results are inconclusive. The value of potassium estimation has been mentioned above.

Studies on other biochemical materials

Such studies, excluding toxicological substances, have been extensively carried out and, because of their wide range of post mortem variations, have been shown in general terms to have little or no forensic importance.

ONSET OF VISIBLE DECOMPOSITION

THERE are two separate processes which cause a body to decompose and disintegrate. These are autolysis and bacterial activity.

Autolysis

This term should be restricted to the softening and eventual liquefaction which occurs in organs, even in the absence of bacteria, for example, the brain or the pancreas. The process is brought about by the cellular destructive activity of tissue enzymes which are liberated after death. Autolysis can be slowed down by the refrigeration of a body or halted by deep freezing conditions.

Bacterial activity

Shortly after death the normal bacterial population of a body begins to invade the surrounding tissues producing gas, the release of tissue fluid and a putrid odour. Most of the bacteria responsible are the anaerobes from the intestinal tract, in particular the *Clostridia*. If the death was caused by a bacterial disease, then the bacterial population is increased and the decomposition is accelerated.

The first sign of bacterial decomposition is a green discolouration of the skin of the lower abdomen, especially in the right lower quadrant, over the caecum. This appears three to four days after death, occasionally as early as 48 hours.

By the end of seven days the discolouration has

spread to involve most of the skin over the abdomen, chest and perhaps the upper parts of the limbs. The skin is green or black, sometimes a deep purple. The skin is now loose, and the superficial layers are easily rubbed off, leaving a soft slippery surface. In the absence of a vital reaction, there is no difficulty in distinguishing 'skin slip' from ante mortem blisters, abrasions or scalds.

During the second week blisters are formed under the skin and there is considerable gas formation. This begins in the gastro-intestinal system and causes great abdominal distension. Blood-stained fluid is forced out of the nose and mouth. Crepitus is present in the skin over the trunk caused by gas-forming bacteria. By the end of the second week there is distension of the soft tissues of the face, breasts, scrotum and penis. From now on, the time scale is blurred. Possibly during the third to the fifth week the hair becomes loosened, the nails can be detached and there is a grotesque appearance to the face in particular and the body in general. An internal examination shows such softening and dissolution of the tissues that a naked eye examination for gross pathological finding is all that can be reasonably achieved. Certain firm fibro-muscle organs show delayed decomposition. These include the uterus and prostate. Their presence may be useful for sex determination of the decomposing remains.

After a number of weeks or perhaps several months, the gas and the liquid contents have drained away and the remaining soft tissues have become considerably reduced in size. The rate of decay is now slowed down. Eventually even the soft tissues largely disappear leaving a skeleton to which the periosteum, tendon insertions and an amorphous fatty mass adhere. The bones then lose these structures after a number of years and the skeleton may remain for hundreds of years, depending on the environmental conditions.

The changes just described are so variable that the timing of the sequence of events cannot be done with any degree of accuracy. There are so many circumstances which will alter the rate of decomposition, that one is advised never to pronounce too readily on how long a body has been lying since death.

When a body begins to decompose in water, the changes that occur depend on the nature and the temperature of the water. The specific gravity of a dead body is only slightly greater than water itself and although it sinks, when gas is formed by the bacteria this alters the specific gravity and allows the body to float. Because the gas is in the chest and abdomen, the usual floating position is one where the trunk is uppermost and the head and limbs hang down.

When a body will surface will depend on the temperature of the water, the depth to which the body sank and whether it is fresh or saltwater. In freshwater in summer, the body could be expected to surface in 4–7 days (the putrefactive processes being similar to a body on land) but in deep seawater in winter it may not surface for two weeks or even longer. Bodies in stagnant warm water with much biological life or in sewage water will decompose more quickly due to animal and bacterial action. Once decomposition has started, and disregarding secondary activity by the marine or freshwater life, the process will follow the same course as for a body on the land.

Special variants of decomposition

There are two important variants or deviants from the normal process of decomposition: *adipocere* and *mummification*. Because of their special significance in forensic medicine each will be described in detail.

Adipocere　One variant of decomposition is adipocere, a word derived from 'adipose' – fatty, and 'cire' – wax. In its early stages it is a soft, yellow greasy material caused by hydrolysis and hydrogenation of the body fat. The formation of adipocere serves to slow or even check the rate of body decomposition. The chemical alteration affects the fat around the internal organs as well as that in the subcutaneous tissues so that the amount of adipocere found is dependent largely on the quantity and distribution of the body fat at the time of death.

　　The texture of adipocere is an indication of its age. After an interval of several weeks, perhaps a few months, the adipocere is soft, greasy and with a strong rancid smell. The texture is similar to margarine. If older, perhaps many months up to a year or two, then the adipocere is white, dry, and easily crumbles, having an earthy or mildly cheesy odour. The body usually, unless quite old, has some elements of each type in the tissues.

　　Early writers believed that adipocere was formed in a damp cold environment, but more recently the reverse has been found to be the case in many bodies.

　　Recent studies show that the humid conditions required for the hydrolysis of fat are found within the body itself. The chief activator is *Clostridium welchii*, an anaerobic bacterium from the intestine, which under warm humid conditions produces lecithinase.

This enzyme assists in the hydrolysis and hydrogenation processes until the temperature drops to about 70°F. The partially completed process is also termed adipocere.

To the pathologist, the presence of adipocere is an indicator that the body has been dead for several weeks, if not many months, depending on its state, but it must be stressed that a precise time cannot be deduced, either from its presence or absence.

The interest in adipocere, especially that occurring immediately under the skin, lies in the fact that it reasonably preserves the outline of the body, especially the face, to allow an identification to be made with some confidence long after death.

Mummification   A second variant of decomposition is mummification. The process is characterized by drying, hardening and shrivelling of the tissues, in particular the skin, and named because of the many dried bodies excavated and uncovered in dry warm regions, notably in Egypt. The normal process of decomposition and putrefaction is slowed down and sometimes halted by a drying-out process which takes place relatively rapidly in a warm atmosphere. Once the change has occurred the skin and many of the soft tissues near the body surface will remain in that state indefinitely, unless attacked by insects, notably the Brown House moth which has a predilection for hair, skin and internal organs.

Whilst a distinction has been drawn between adipocere and mummification, in practice this can be less easily made than has been implied above. The overlap between the two conditions can be considerable, suggesting that the drying process has been slow. This has allowed the adipocere process to begin until the

63

essential humidity is lost by drying and the mummification process takes over.

Mummification of a body of a newly born child (viable or non-viable) is the most frequent example seen and in temperate regions it should take several months to develop fully. Partial mummification of the skin of fingers, toes, or ears may occur independently of the rest of the body, and this may be seen as early as four to six weeks after death.

A special form of mummification is seen in the well-preserved bodies discovered in peat bogs throughout Northern Europe. Many have been estimated by pollen analysis, radio-carbon dating and circumstantial artefactual evidence to have been buried about 2000 years previously. The appearance of the skin is soft, leathery and very dark brown. The bones have had the minerals leached out and are therefore very pliable.

Preservation, to the extent that considerable features still remain identifiable, is explained by the cold, airless, acid environment in which humic and tannic acids act on the tissues to preserve them.

FORENSIC ENTOMOLOGY

THIS is an area almost overlooked by forensic pathologists, but which under the guidance of an entomologist is worthy of some basic study. With practice, the study of the insects which visit a cadaver can give some reliable data as to the time of death. Entomology is particularly useful when bodies are discovered in a fairly advanced state of putrefraction.

Insects visit a body, whether human or animal, in successive waves. The first arrivals are the necrophagous varieties which come primarily to feed on the corpse and to lay their eggs. These include the family of flies, or *Diptera*, amongst which are the Common Bluebottle (*Calliphora erythrocephala*), the Green-bottle (*Lucilia caesar* or *Lucilia sericata*) and the Common Housefly (*Musca domestica*).

The second invaders feed on the first group, important among these are several varieties of beetle (*Coleoptera*). Next come the omnivorous insects, the wasps, ants, etc. (*Hymenoptera*). Lastly arrive a miscellany of insects who come for shelter or warmth from the decomposing body.

Common bluebottle (Calliphora erythrocephala)

This large fly is of considerable value to the forensic pathologist because it visits the body so soon after death. The eggs are laid readily on tissues which are fresh – less commonly when they have started to decompose. The maximum number of eggs laid by a single fly is of the order of 2000. They are deposited in groups of about 150 during the hours of daylight, at the edges of orifices, such as the nose, mouth and eyes, or close to wounds. The eggs are laid within a day or two of death.

In summer the eggs hatch in approximately 8 to 14 hours, producing white maggots. These quickly invade the adjacent tissues, often to a great depth, liquefying the tissues as they advance.

The maggot (larva) undergoes three stages of growth, each ending in a moult. Each stage is termed an instar, which is the time between two successive castings of the cuticle or outer skin. The mature larva then leaves the body to pupate. This occurs during the night, some distance from the food supply in the soil, in clothing or body wrappings, from which stage a fully developed fly emerges.

The duration of each stage, under average conditions, is reasonably constant; they are accelerated by heat, moisture and an ample food supply; and slowed by adverse conditions.

From the laying of the egg to the developed fly, the time taken is between 21 and 24 days.

The stages are as follows:

1 Deposition of the eggs = 1–2 days after death has occurred.
2 Eggs hatching to 1st larva = 8–14 hours later.
3 1st larva to 2nd larva = 8–14 hours later.
4 2nd larva to 3rd larva = 2–3 days later.
5 3rd larva to pupa = 6–7 days later.
6 Pupa to fly = 12–13 days later.

This knowledge has been applied in estimating the time of death in several cases of interest. For example, in the Ruxton Murders (Glaister and Brash) the larvae were identified as third instar larvae of *Calliphora*. The finding proved of corroborative value.

Greenbottle (Lucilia caesar or Lucilia sericata)

The life histories of these flies are similar in all respects to that of the Bluebottle.

Common Housefly (Musca domestica)

The younger instars are very similar to those of the *Calliphora* and *Lucilia* but the fully grown larvae of

Musca are much smaller than the other two.

The female lays about 150 eggs at a time mainly in body discharges rather than directly on the dead body.

From the laying of the egg to the developed fly takes between 13–15 days.

Distinguishing the three types of larvae

The larva of *Musca* is distinguished from *Calliphora* and *Lucilia* by examining microscopically the stigmata, or breathing pores, at the posterior end.

In *Musca* the spiracles in the stigma are convoluted but in the other two flies the spiracles are straight. At the anterior end of the larva an examination of the mandible will distinguish *Calliphora* from *Lucilia*. In *Calliphora* the mandibular jaw-hook has an additional horizontal process (the accessory oral sclerite) being absent in *Lucilia*.

For evidential purposes in any legal proceedings, the assistance of an entomologist would be sought, if at all possible.

POST MORTEM ARTEFACTS

Animal-induced

Bodies found in sandy locations, especially in the summer, will be invaded by a variety of insects such as ants and beetles. They will produce extensive superficial tissue damage which resemble abrasions. These injuries might be thought to have been produced by dragging through the sand or over rough ground. The lack of linear patterns should be sufficient to exclude dragging injuries.

In more covered places, rats, mice, dogs and foxes may feed on bodies especially in winter when normal food supplies have been exhausted. Animals when ravenous have been known to destroy large areas of a body.

Buzzards, crows and other birds have been seen around a body and they can execute considerable damage, rendering a body almost to a skeleton in a few days, depending very much on the time of the year and their feeding requirements.

When a body is found in water there are numerous invaders which may cause extensive damage to the soft tissues. Crabs, shrimps and other crustaceans, some fish and sea-feeding birds are the common culprits but in tropical water there are many others including turtles and sharks.

All these possibilities must be kept in mind and a close examination of the edge of the injuries may reveal characteristic teeth, beak or claw marks.

Pathologist-induced

In removing the throat organs care must be exercised so as not to fracture the segments of the thyroid cartilage or the hyoid bone. Failure to recognize that he has caused the damage may lead the pathologist to an erroneous opinion of an ante mortem fracture.

In elderly debilitated persons there may be unusual fragility of the bones, especially the ribs. Rough handling or undue pressure on the chest may cause them to fracture, and without due care a wrong interpretation will be placed on the finding.

Undue haste or inability to see clearly may produce a knife cut or tissue damage which may not be appreciated at once. Failure to recognize his own clumsiness may cause a false interpretation to be given to the damage done.

Clinician-induced

Vigorous resuscitative care or diagnostic techniques in the ante mortem period may leave a series of bruises, abrasions, therapeutic injection marks and other tissue damage. To the pathologist unaccustomed to these signs they may be misinterpreted. Unusual bruises found on a body of a child have given rise prematurely to thoughts of child abuse. If in doubt as to what an unusual mark is, the pathologist should request the attendance of the clinician to explain it.

A situation in which this is important is when a victim of a stabbing is admitted to the hospital seriously ill and dies after surgery. At autopsy other stab wounds for diagnostic purposes or for therapy are frequently seen along with the fatal wound. Worse still is the case where a surgeon has enlarged a true stab wound, thus virtually destroying the evidence. The surgeon must be present at the time of the autopsy to identify his wounds and to explain his actions to the satisfaction of the pathologist.

Embalmer-induced

The process of embalming a body is increasingly in

demand and it is essential if the body is to be transported out of the country. On occasion it is carried out before an autopsy is performed.

The initial stages are easily identified because the incisions are made over major blood vessels in the neck, elbow and upper thigh. The later stages consist of passing a trochar into the cavities and the larger organs. The procedure causes extensive and bizarre puncture wounds and will release blood, urine, gastric contents, bile and other fluids into the cavities. Apart from the direct effect of the embalming fluid on the organs, this post mortem trauma may make the interpretation of findings rather difficult.

Machine-induced

This problem is the most difficult of all to interpret. Bodies in water can be severely mutilated by passing ships. Apart from the screw, which can reap extensive havoc on a body, there are many underwater projections on modern ships which can produce lacerations and fractures.

In road traffic accidents there is the problem of a body having been knocked down by one vehicle only to be struck or run over by a following vehicle. There is always difficulty in trying to distinguish primary from secondary injuries.

Other areas of interest include industrial accidents involving moving parts of machinery, high speed accidents as with railway or aircraft accidents. All cases are difficult cases. The pathologist will always welcome help from any direction, both expert and non-expert, before expressing an opinion as to the cause of the injuries. Once made it is often difficult to retract it and replace it with a plausible alternative.

In studying post mortem changes and the variety of pathological findings that present themselves it is of paramount importance that those professionals who have an interest in the results do not too readily arrive at a conclusion. It pays to be cautious. Always remember to maintain an open mind until all the facts are known, recognizing that there are few scientific certainties in post mortem appearances.

REFERENCES

Brown, A. & Marshall, T.K. (1974), *For. Sci.*, **4**, 125.

Coe, J.I. (1974), *J. For. Sci.*, **19**, 13.

Glaister, J. & Brash, J.C. (1937), *Medico-Legal Aspects of the Ruxton Case*, Livingtone, Edinburgh.

Knight, B. (1987), *Legal Aspects of Medical Practice*, 4th edn, Churchill Livingstone, London, p. 121.

Marshall, T.K. & Hoare, P.E. (1962), *J. For. Sci.*, **7**, 56.

3 THE POST MORTEM EXAMINATION

THE procedure whereby the pathologist anatomically removes all the organs from a body for the purposes of a pathological examination is expressed in a number of ways. These include: an autopsy, a necropsy, a medico-legal dissection and a post mortem examination. The descriptions are used interchangeably, but it is the latter term which is the one most widely used by police officers, lawyers, pathologists and the general public, to the extent that in general conversation it is frequently abbreviated to the letters – PM.

It has to be understood that the external examination and the subsequent dissection of a body is the only conclusive means of discovering the cause of death, in so far as the mode of death leaves behind sufficient evidence of the pathological or toxicological processes involved. The autopsy allows a study to be made of all the stages through which a healthy person passes until his death.

A post mortem examination is a carefully planned, unhurried dissection of each of the tissues and organs, in order that the process of dying can be scientifically investigated in a logical, step-wise manner. It follows, therefore, that it cannot be regarded as a mere disembowelling process, performed in a rapid rather casual manner. If that were the case, nothing would be achieved. Throughout the entire operation there must be maintained by all persons involved a proper, professional respect, first towards the body itself and to those relatives to whom it belongs, and second, to those persons whose interests are linked to the results which the pathologist is able to uncover.

REQUEST FOR A POST MORTEM EXAMINATION

THE request may arise from a number of sources, but the nature of the autopsy will fall into one of four classes.

Hospital autopsy

If the deceased had been treated medically or surgically in a hospital or a nursing home, the consultant concerned may request an autopsy, after he has obtained the consent of the deceased's nearest relatives, or of some other person having the right of possession of the body. The post mortem examination is requested for the following purposes:

(a) to establish the true cause of death;*
(b) to enable the doctor to correlate the signs, symptoms and his clinical diagnosis with the pathological findings revealed at the autopsy;
(c) to enable the physician or surgeon to evalu-

ate the effectiveness of his treatment by therapy or by surgery;

(d) to allow an opportunity for the doctor to study the natural course of disease processes;

(e) to form an important part of the undergraduate and postgraduate education programme;

(f) to allow the removal of certain organs and tissues for transplantation purposes, under the terms of the Human Tissue Act, 1961.

Forensic autopsy

The medico-legal post mortem examination is undertaken in accordance with existing laws of each individual nation, having due regard for the need to protect the interests of the state and the general public. To this end, before a pathologist is able to carry out the work, it is the permission of the state, rather than the permission of private individuals, that must be given. In the UK this is granted by Her Majesty's Coroners in England, Wales and Northern Ireland, or by a sheriff's warrant, on application by the procurator-fiscal for the area, in Scotland. The interests of the state will override any private person's objection to the performance of an autopsy, and furthermore, will set aside a private person's right to

---

* It is unlawful for a doctor in the UK to withhold issuing a death certificate, until the deceased's relatives first grant permission for a post mortem examination, solely on the grounds that he must have an autopsy performed, to enable him to complete and then issue the death certificate.

If the doctor is unable to issue a death certificate because of ignorance as to a reasonable cause of death, then he has no alternative but to refer the matter to the legal authorities, who will then order a medico-legal investigation.

accept and dispose of the body, until after the results of the medico-legal autopsy have been made known and there is no further interest in the body itself.

The post mortem dissection will be performed by an appointed pathologist for the following reasons:

(a) to establish as far as possible, the identity of the person or his remains;

(b) to determine, as accurately as possible, the cause and the manner of death;

(c) to estimate the time of death;

(d) to assist in establishing the place where death occurred;

(e) to collect, identify and preserve both biological and non-biological material for evidential purposes at any subsequent enquiry or trial;

(f) to distinguish death due to natural causes from unnatural causes;

(g) to provide the documented facts in an acceptable form for the coroner, the procurator-fiscal, the prosecuting and defending lawyers, the police, the families of the deceased and their legal representatives and to all other persons who may have a need for, or a right to, such medical investigation.

Cremation autopsy

Before granting permission for a cremation to proceed, the medical referee of a crematorium may request a pathologist to perform a post mortem examination on the deceased. The referee may, if he is also a pathologist, carry out the autopsy himself. Although the request for such an examination is not frequently made, it does remove any doubts that the referee may have regarding the death. These will have arisen from the manner in which the cremation forms have been completed by the medical practitioners. As an alternative the medical referee may refer the entire matter to the coroner or the procurator-fiscal who, in turn, will arrange for his own medico-legal examination to be carried out.

Private autopsy

Occasionally, a request for an autopsy will come from the relatives of the deceased, where the death occurred at home or abroad, or in a place, not being a hospital. It may or may not be with the persuasion of the family practitioner. The reasons are often not entirely clear, but nevertheless there is a sincere wish to know for themselves the true nature of their relative's illness. It can only be performed after a death certificate has been issued and the death registered, and of course there must be no question of any irregularities concerning the death. Rarely, the deceased himself may have expressed a wish either in life before witnesses or as a codicil to his will, that upon his death a post mortem examination be performed for the purposes of medical research.

THE MEDICO-LEGAL AUTOPSY

THE main requirements of a forensic post mortem examination are that:

(a) the pathologist appointed for the occasion must be fully experienced in routine, non-legal autopsies and have received adequate instruction to perform a medico-legal autopsy;

(b) all the information gathered by the pathologist be suitably recorded at the time of the examination, or shortly thereafter;

(c) a factual, complete and objective report with appropriate unbiased conclusions based on his findings be made available to the individual parties.

In many jurisdictions throughout Europe, the post mortem examination is performed by a single pathologist, but in Scotland the examination is frequently undertaken by two pathologists jointly. This is essential when the facts of the autopsy form part of the evidence in any subsequent trial or enquiry. Under the Law of Evidence in Scotland, all material evidence must be corroborated if it is to be rendered admissible in court. The names of the two pathologists appointed for the autopsy appear on the sheriff's warrant. Whilst in practice one person performs the dissection and the other records the findings, the eventual agreed report is signed by both pathologists.

Preliminary procedures

Before the autopsy can be started there are a number of important matters which have to be considered:

1 Everybody who has any interest whatsoever in the fact that a post mortem examination is to take place should be fully informed well in advance as to the time and place where it will be performed. This will allow those who wish to be present, or represented, the opportunity to learn the results or to be party to the discussions on the case.

2   The necessary legal authority to perform the dissection must have been granted to the pathologist. This may be through the coroner's officer or at the request of the procurator-fiscal.

3   The formalities of identifying the deceased person must have been observed. This may be done by the accompanying police officer or, as in Scotland, by two persons who knew the deceased in life. In the latter case their names, addresses and relationships to the deceased require to be formally recorded.

4   What information there is regarding the deceased should be made available to the pathologist by the police or by the legal authorities.

5   The services of a properly trained mortuary attendant should be readily available to help with the autopsy, both before and after the actual removal and dissection of the organs.

If any one of these matters be deficient, it would be prudent for the pathologist and the police to postpone the autopsy until the situation has been rectified.

There is one important problem to be faced, although thankfully it is one which presents itself less often than in former years, and that concerns the place where the autopsy is to be carried out. The notion of a post mortem examination to some people, and that includes some members of the police, is still that of a messy dissection performed in some out-of-the-way place deficient in many of the modern facilities. It was not unknown for pathologists, often relatively recently, to be offered space in an outbuilding, a former police garage, old stabling at a small cottage hospital, or, as in one notable case, an extension to the dog-pound, with a common, open, inadequate drainage system.

There is no excuse today for the pathologist to be asked to work in such primitive, sub-standard conditions. If offered such facilities, he is justified in firmly refusing to accept them. To accept would be unprofessional and would carry a serious health risk. Furthermore it would probably be unproductive with regard to his eventual conclusions based on his work.

The police must accept responsibility and make proper arrangements to have the body transported to a properly equipped mortuary, where opportunities are available for a complete inspection of the body in a good light. There must be reasonable facilities to hand for a comprehensive post mortem dissection. In addition, there must be sufficient space for the police photographer or video team and the forensic scientists to work as well as the pathologist, without the prospects of everybody getting in each other's way.

REMOVAL OF CLOTHING FROM A BODY

MORTUARY attendants, police, ambulance personnel and others who may be on hand when a body arrives at the mortuary are sometimes unsure as to whether they should remove the clothing before transferring the body either to the cold storage room, or on to the dissecting table. This is a matter where the pathologist concerned must give clear and precise instructions. He must decide what procedure he wishes to be followed, bearing in mind possible questions in court at a later date on this particular point. Only by the adoption of some plan will confusion and mistakes be avoided. In general terms, when the autopsy is related to the perpetration of a serious crime, or where there exists an inordinate degree of suspicion regarding the cause of death, then the body should be left in the clothes in which it arrived at the mortuary.

Undressing the body will then take place in the presence of the pathologist. On the other hand, when death occurred in circumstances not regarded as being suspicious, then there is no reason for the body not to be undressed and prepared for subsequent dissection.

A suggested procedure to be followed in those cases in which there is some degree of suspicion is as follows.

The body, while still clothed, should be photographed both in full-length and in close-up views, paying particular attention to any obvious wounds or injuries. At this stage the exposed parts should not be cleaned in order to make the photograph more agreeable: the amount and distribution of blood or dirt may prove later to be of invaluable assistance. Take sufficient photographs – it is often impossible to repeat them at a later time.

As each item of clothing and jewellery is removed, it must be recorded and carefully labelled and signed for identification purposes. The pathologist must also sign each label. It is preferable to use brown paper bags rather than thin plastic bags, because there is then less likelihood of condensation inside the bag which may interfere with the laboratory investigations. If the clothing is wet or heavily blood-stained it should be allowed to dry in the air before being sealed in the paper bag. This will minimize putrefaction and disintegration.

The indiscriminate use of scissors for cutting off clothing from rigid bodies should be avoided. Any cuts or tears that have to be made must be made well away from areas of special interest, and the action taken must be recorded. It is always useful to make a general inspection of each item before it is packaged, because then an overall impression of the number, sites and sizes of any holes present can be made, but defer any *detailed* examination until the items can be seen in the laboratory by the forensic scientist.

All items removed from the body must be handed over to the police, whose responsibility it is to label each item and despatch them to the legal authorities and to the laboratory. They are also responsible for their eventual safe-keeping before a trial.

The face should now be washed and prepared for the formal identification by relatives.

Further duties

Now that the body is nude, any further wounds, previously unseen, should be photographed.

The remainder of the body should be carefully washed, paying particular attention to the wounds. Any adherent foreign material should be left in place, at this stage, unless the pathologist directs otherwise. Head wounds should be exposed by shaving away the surrounding hair.

Further photographs should now be taken, including where possible a small scale or ruler to indicate the size of any close-up views. Remember that these photographs may well be on display at any subsequent trial.

The removal of samples of head and pubic hair should now be done followed by swab samples taken from the mouth, vagina and anus. In this way contamination by other body fluids will be avoided. In certain cases, e.g. in sexual murder, these laboratory samples should be taken before the body is washed, to avoid contact with soapy water and disinfectant fluid. The hair should be pulled out rather than cut off, so as to obtain the entire hair for examination. Any foreign material adherent to the body should be removed. Nail scrapings or clippings should also be taken and these with all the specimens must be placed in separately labelled containers. After a handgun has been fired, powder residue may be detected on the hands by the use of specialized laboratory techniques. If they are to be used, then, from the outset of the autopsy, the hands should be protected from contamination by covering them with plastic or paper bags until the scientist arrives.

THE EXTERNAL EXAMINATION OF THE BODY

BEFORE the dissection can be started, there must be a full and systematic external examination of the body, and this should include relevant comments on the build, height and weight, as well as the state of nutrition, sexual development, the presence and extent of post mortem lividity and the degree of muscular rigidity. The colour of the eyes and hair, the nature of any bodily deformities or abnormalities, e.g. scars and tattoo marks, should all be carefully noted and recorded.

An inspection of the skin for petechial or pinpoint haemorrhages away from areas showing post mortem lividity may suggest an asphyxial death. Blisters on the limbs or trunk may indicate burning, or barbiturate intoxication. It may also indicate early decomposition of the body. A pronounced skin rash in a child may be a pointer to a bacterial infection, such as meningococcal meningitis, or a dirty unwashed skin, perhaps light brown in colour, may indicate a person's state of living before death. Above all the presence of any wounds or injuries, however small, must be measured, described and noted down.

There are certain areas of the body which require particular attention and these are listed separately.

Wounds in the *scalp* may be easily missed in a thick head of hair. Often they are not discovered until after the scalp has been stripped away from the skull. If however, injuries are suspected, the hair must be shaved off so that the area can be clearly seen.

The *eyelids and the surrounding soft tissues* may be infiltrated by blood and yet not show any significant tissue swelling. Often this appearance affects both eyes to an equal extent. This has a special significance in that two 'black eyes' may be the first indication of a fracture to the base of the skull. This is usually through the orbital plates which lie immediately above each eye. The haemorrhage produced tracks forwards, by way of the peri-orbital loose tissues, to appear on the front of the face.

The *eyes* should be examined for corneal or lens opacities. The presence of a cataract in the eyes of a person knocked down in a road traffic accident may be important in trying to establish how the death occurred. The degree of pupil dilatation and any dissimilarity in the two eyes must be noted.

On turning back the eyelids, the *conjunctivae* and in particular the fornices should be examined for the presence of petechial haemorrhages, for these may be the only external signs that death was due to asphyxia.

The *ears and the nose* should be examined for

haemorrhage, indicating fractures to the base of the skull and the nasal bones. Do remember however that blood from a facial injury may run down into the ears, creating a false impression that the blood originated from the ears.

An inspection of the *lips, the frenum, the gums and the teeth or dentures* at this stage, may reveal injuries which may not be so obvious at a later time. They might even be overlooked. The tongue will be examined more easily later, after its removal, but at this point just note its position relative to the teeth. Is it being bitten or trapped between the teeth?

The assistance of a dental surgeon may be required in matters concerning the *teeth, jaws and mouth*, and if this is the case, it is wise to consult him before going any further. He may wish to make his examination at this time, rather than waiting until after the mouth and neck structures have been removed.

The *skin of the front of the neck* must be examined with care to determine whether bruises, fingernail abrasions, ligature marks and bite marks are present. Special attention is required in infants, when post mortem refrigeration frequently hardens the subcutaneous fat. This makes normal skin folds appear as excessively deep creases. They can easily be misinterpreted as ligature marks if their true nature is not recognized. The head should be extended well back, preferably over a block of wood or some similar object to expose this area. The neck must be examined before the start of the dissection: it is impossible to reconstruct the tissues adequately once the first incision has been made. At the same time an assessment of the mobility of the neck should be made. Abnormal mobility may well indicate a fractured neck.

An inspection and palpation of the *surface of the chest* may show an abnormal flattening resulting from a severe crushing injury. The upper part of the chest is a good site for the presence of petechial haemorrhages resulting from the blockage of very small blood vessels by fat droplets, released after extensive bone damage.

Any *distension of the abdomen* should be looked for, but swelling due to the presence of massive tumours or ascitic fluid is much more frequently seen in hospital practice than in forensic medicine.

The *surfaces of the hands and arms* must never be forgotten. Much useful information can be obtained from the presence and the site of abrasions and lacerations, the state of the fingernails and the presence and position of defence wounds. Do not make this a cursory examination just because the fingers and wrists are in full flexion due to rigor mortis. To examine adequately the palm and fingers, forcibly hyperflex the wrist when the fingers will be seen to extend of their own accord.

Note the site, number and area of any injection marks, having in mind the possibility of drug dependence. Note too, any orthopaedic abnormalities to fingers or thumbs such as might follow industrial accidents. If electrocution is suspected as being the cause of death, search diligently on and between the fingers for a small, often quite tiny, electrical mark.

The *lower limbs* should be examined, especially if ankle oedema is present, and the more common local causes such as deep venous thrombosis, varicose ulceration, peripheral arterial occlusive disease and secondary cancer in the groin are worth considering, apart from any general circulatory and renal causes.

The *external genitalia, the perineum and the anus*

should not be overlooked. Whilst details for examining these areas are properly reserved for the chapter on sexual offences, it is often rewarding for the pathologist to make a superficial examination at each autopsy. It is sound practice for all interested parties to consider a sexual motive or at least a sexual component to be present in every suspicious female death.

The value of *an X-ray examination of a body* is often underestimated. All too frequently it is simply forgotten. Radiological studies can be of great value in locating foreign objects such as bullets, as well as helping to locate fractures, anatomical deformities and dental and orthopaedic surgical appliances.

THE INTERNAL EXAMINATION OF THE BODY

A POST mortem examination must include the inspection, removal and dissection of all internal organs of the body, although the apparent cause of death may be found in just one organ or system. It is possible that evidence contributory to the cause of death will be found elsewhere in the body. Frequently, outside observers to a post mortem examination express surprise that the pathologist, having quickly established a reasonable, or even a certain, cause of death, then continues to dissect all the remaining organs which have no apparent bearing on the cause of death. The importance of a complete internal examination of the body cannot be too strongly stressed, as an inadvertent failure to do so may invalidate the subsequent medical report, or at least expose its contents to question.

There is no 'right' way to perform an autopsy, nor indeed is there a standard way; each pathologist will discover the technique that suits him best, and then adopt it as his routine method. Likewise his selected procedure will not be rigidly adhered to, for when an abnormal situation arises he must be flexible enough to adopt some other technique, however unusual.

Primary incisions

A commonly used method consists of a simple mid-line incision, beginning about 5cm below the point of the chin to end just above the pubic bone, avoiding the umbilicus. The soft tissues are reflected from off the rib cage as far out as the mid-axillary line. The abdominal incision is deepened to open the abdominal cavity.

A second method is a modification of the first in that the neck structures are more easily exposed by a Y-shaped incision. A separate incision is made on each side of the neck beginning 3cm behind the lobe of each ear. The two incisions run downwards and medially to meet at the upper border of the breast bone from which point a single mid-line incision continues down to the pubis. The V-shaped flap of skin in the front of the neck is reflected upwards as far as the line of the lower jaw. This results in a good exposure of all the structures in the neck.

A third method, and one greatly favoured in North America, comprises a broad Y-shaped incision but placed lower down on the body, so that the arms of the Y begin at the tips of the shoulders and they meet in the centre of the chest. The method has the advantage of completely concealing the suture line when the body is dressed for viewing by relatives, but it has the time-consuming disadvantage of requiring the pathologist to reflect a very large flap of skin from the mid-sternum up to the lower jaw.

Regional examinations

(i) *The head* With the back of the head resting on a wooden block the scalp is incised transversely across the vault to end behind each ear lobe. If the second method of primary incision described above, is used, then the scalp incision will join up with the neck lines on each side. The scalp is then separated from the skull anteriorly as far as the level of the eyebrows, and posteriorly as far as the upper part of the neck. This manoeuvre enables the scalp and the adjacent temporal muscles to be examined for bruises. They are much more obvious on this side of the scalp than down among the hair. The vault of the skull is now ready for removal by the use of a hand-saw or an electric autopsy saw. The usual method is to produce a circular cut begining well above the level of the eyebrows in the front and posteriorly through the occiput. With the vault removed, the outer meningeal layer, the dura mater, is removed, during which time the presence of any blood in the extradural and subdural spaces is looked for.

After the brain has been removed, the dura is stripped from the base of the skull to expose any fractures. In an adult this is easily done, but it is a difficult task in an infant; nevertheless it should not be overlooked.

(ii) *The neck* Because of the close proximity of several vital structures in the neck, both to the skin surface as well as to each other, injuries to the neck structures assume an important role in forensic medicine. For example, asphyxia due to one of several different causes may easily be missed unless a careful dissection of the neck organs is undertaken. It is necessary to place a support under the shoulders, with the head well back, to get a good exposure of the front of the neck. Dissecting outwards on either side of the mid-line primary incision and starting under the lower jaw will release the tongue, larynx, pharynx, oesophagus, trachea, carotid vessels, vagus nerves and the thyroid gland as a single entity.

A useful and frequently helpful modification can be made in those cases where, from the history of the circumstances of the death, bruises and other injuries to the neck are anticipated. By the use of the second primary incision, the 'Y-shaped' incision, the skin is lifted up from the neck structures. These structures are now left untouched until after the contents of the thorax have first been removed by cutting across them at the root of the neck and second, the intracranial contents have also been removed. This allows any blood remaining in the neck vessels to drain away in either direction. The dissection of the neck structures can now proceed in a 'bloodless field', and any free blood seen lying in the neck tissues must have arrived there in life, and not by the technique of the pathologist.

(iii) *The thorax*   After the skin and the chest muscles have been separated from the ribs, the chest cavity can be opened. In young bodies this is done by dividing the costal cartilages on either side with a knife, but in older bodies where the costal cartilages have become calcified, this is best done with a pair of rib shears or a hand-saw. Together with the sternum the central block of bone and cartilage can be removed, allowing the chest contents to be inspected. Once the subclavian arteries at the root of the neck are divided, and provided that there are no firm adhesions on the surface of the lungs, binding the lungs to the rib cage, the trachea, oesophagus and aorta can all be pulled forwards and downwards thus raising the entire thoracic viscera out of the chest cavity. When the aorta, the inferior vena cava and the oesophagus are cut across at the level of the diaphragm, the contents of the thoracic cavity can now be removed for a detailed examination.

There are two special situations where it is desirable that the pathologist examine certain thoracic organs before their removal:

(a) When a pulmonary blood clot embolus is suspected, the right ventricle and the pulmonary trunk should be opened *in situ*, and their contents examined.

(b) When a pulmonary air embolus is suspected, an incision is made through the parietal pericardium. The pericardial sac is held open by forceps and the sac is filled with water. The right ventricle is held under the water with gentle pressure and an incision into the ventricle is made *in situ*. If air is present in the right ventricle or pulmonary trunk it will bubble up through the water. The method requires care both with the operation and with the interpretation of the results.

(iv) *The abdomen* The abdominal cavity should always be inspected carefully before any attempt is made to remove the organs. This will include a search for adhesions, free-lying fluid, the presence of peritonitis, or other pathological entities whose presence may be missed when contaminated with blood or when the organs are removed.

To remove the abdominal organs, one begins by removing the small and large intestines. At the upper end the jejunum is ligated close to its junction with the duodenum and then cut across. At the lower end the rectum is ligated in its middle portion and divided below the ligature.

The remaining abdominal organs are removed either separately, in groups or *en bloc*. Lastly the contents of the pelvis are isolated from the walls of the pelvis and cut across in the bottom of the pelvic cavity.

(v) *The skeleton* When all the organs have been removed, the cranial, thoracic, abdominal and pelvic cavities are cleaned out ready for inspection. The base of the skull, the vertebral column, the ribs and the several parts of the pelvis are palpated and inspected. If the circumstances warrant it, the long bones of the limbs are exposed and removed, the upper vertebral column is separated from the base of the skull and a thin sliver of bone is removed from the anterior surface of the vertebral column.

Special procedures

The foregoing details were intended to help those who have not had an opportunity of being present when an uncomplicated autopsy was performed. There are several special procedures which are undertaken, although the number of occasions when they will be required may be limited, and these are now described in a little more detail.

(i) *Removal of the female pelvic organs* The soft tissues behind the pubis and the attachments of the pelvic organs to the pelvis and the vertebral column are freed as mentioned above, but now the urethra, vagina and rectum are not cut across. The thighs are widely separated to give ready access to the vulva, perineum and anus. An oval incision is made through the skin beginning above the clitoris and passing downwards on either side of the labia majora to end behind the anus. From the upper end of this oval incision the knife is passed under the pubic bone into the pelvic cavity. The deep incision is continued round the inside of the bones forming the outlet to the pelvis until all the pelvic organs and the external genitalia are freed and can be removed as one specimen from out of the pelvic cavity.

The purpose of the manoeuvre allows the pathologist to open up the entire genital tract so that a thorough search for any injuries can be made more easily.

(ii) *Removal of the male genital organs and pelvic organs* Each testis and spermatic cord can be exposed and removed by separating the loose subcutaneous tissue between the skin and the inguinal ligament. The scrotal contents can then be emptied on either side.

To remove the entire urethra, the pelvic contents are freed as described above, but the urethra is not divided. The original abdominal skin incision is continued over the pubis and along the dorsal surface of the penis as far as the glans. The shaft of the penis is freed from the skin, and all the loose tissue under the arch of the pubis. The penis is then pushed under the symphysis pubis into the pelvic cavity where it can be removed, still attached, along with the remaining pelvic organs. After opening the bladder the dissection can continue along the entire length of the urethra.

(iii) *Block dissection of the calf muscles*   In every case where a pulmonary embolus is discovered, or even suspected, it is necessary to determine the site of origin. In most cases this will be found in the deep veins of the calf muscles. The best way to examine the veins is to remove the muscles *en bloc* after which they can be serially sliced or dissected out. A longitudinal incision is made on the front of the lower leg and the skin separated from the muscle planes by passing round to the back of the leg on each side inside the skin and passing under the tibia and fibula. It is most unsatisfactory to make deep horizontal cuts at random through the back of the calf into the muscle groups. A negative finding by this means is valueless.

(iv) *Removal of spinal cord*   It is not often the case that the spinal cord need be removed in medico-legal practice, but in certain cases of head injury, dislocation of the neck, crushing injuries of the neck, strychnine poisoning and certain viral infections, the procedure assumes an important role.

There are two approaches that can be made, but the easier is made from the front of the body after all the internal organs have been removed. A series of lateral cuts on each side of the vertebral bodies is made with the electric autopsy saw, allowing the front of the bones to be removed, thereby exposing the spinal canal and within it the spinal cord surrounded by the dura. Once the dural attachments and the emerging nerves have been carefully cut the spinal cord can be removed.

THE REFRIGERATION OF BODIES

ALMOST all mortuaries are now equipped with facilities for storing bodies at a variety of low temperatures in specially designed chambers. This has the effect of slowing down the onset of rigor mortis if the body has been inserted shortly after death. Similarly if cooled at a later stage, the process of putrefaction is retarded. An immediate sign of a refrigerated body is the presence of reddish blotches on the dependent regions, both on the surface of the body and sometimes on the organs. The bright reddish colouration must not be interpreted as signs of carbon monoxide poisoning, cyanide poisoning or death due to exposure and hypothermia.

THE EFFECTS OF EMBALMING

THE practice of preserving a body from natural decomposition by embalming is performed infrequently in the UK, although the process is more frequently carried out in other countries, for example in North America. The process involves injecting through the large arteries of the body a preserving fluid, containing formaldehyde, methyl alcohol and a colouring agent. It is important to remember that whilst the process does not significantly interfere with any subsequent post mortem dissection, the removal of any specimens for bacteriological, virological and toxicological studies will be made very difficult, if not impossible.

THE POST MORTEM EXAMINATION

EXHUMATIONS

It is sometimes necessary, where the cause of death is disputed, to exhume a body for the purpose of settling the dispute. An exhumation order is usually made where a crime has been suspected or, in civil matters, for example in matters of life insurance.

In England and Wales, at common law, a coroner may order an exhumation for the purposes of inquisition. For other purposes, consent must be obtained from the Home Secretary under Section 25, Burial Act, 1857.

In Scotland, a sheriff, after petition, may grant a warrant. In a civil case, a petition is presented either to the sheriff, or to the Court of Session by the party desiring the exhumation.

In both countries the relatives are given an opportunity for raising any objections in the civil cases. After the hearing the authority is granted to the medical practitioners and the graveyard authorities to have the body exhumed.

Certain precautions must be adopted. First, the grave must be identified by the graveyard authorities and the grave digger. Then the coffin should be identified by the undertaker. In any recent interment it is an unpleasant operation and one fraught with danger, particularly in the case of a person who is suspected of having died from an infectious disease.

It is usually found to be most convenient to make the examination in the early morning, before the cemetery is open to the public, in order to obtain some measure of privacy. The grave is surrounded by some screening material and the whole operation is conducted under police supervision.

Soil samples from above, below and at the sides of

95

the coffin are taken together with some of the water in the coffin and sent for analysis. A full autopsy is performed, as far as the tissues will allow, and where necessary toxicological studies are carried out.

At the conclusion of the exhumation a formal legal enquiry will be held after which the coroner or the procurator-fiscal will issue an order for re-burial.

4   DISPOSAL OF THE DEAD

THE shock and stress of a sudden death in the family results in bereaved members turning to any professional person, close at hand, for advice and assistance. In this chapter we shall consider some medico-legal problems to which the professional should address himself.

In general terms, it is unlawful to dispose of a body until its identity has been established, the cause of death has been ascertained and the death has been registered. These points need amplification.

IDENTIFICATION

THE problems surrounding the identification of an individual body, or part of it, are discussed elsewhere. Nevertheless, despite these measures, a body may persistently lie unidentified. The body is then retained in a suitable refrigerated place, whilst nationwide enquiries may be made using all sections of the media, and an opportunity given for the general public to approach the police regarding missing relatives. After a reasonable length of time, and with little or no hope of success in establishing the identity, the body is then released for burial, but not for cremation, as 'A person of unknown identity'. The responsibility usually lies with the social work department of the local authority.

CAUSE OF DEATH

FROM time to time the forensic pathologist has had to admit that he has been unable to determine the cause of death, despite intensive and wide-ranging investigations. Given that often he has only a disintegrating body, or one undergoing advanced decomposition to work on, it is perhaps not too surprising that he is unable to state the cause of death. However, when the cause of death in a recently deceased body cannot be ascertained, there is almost a sense of embarrassment on the part of all concerned.

Example Two elderly sisters, living together, were both found recently dead, side by side, on the bedroom floor, close to their double bed. It was a comfortable, all-electric flat, but with no signs of faulty equipment. Alcohol or other drugs were not detected in the bodies. The only pathological findings were long-standing heart disease and chronic bronchitis, neither disease being sufficiently advanced to give rise to a double sudden death.

After extensive pathological studies, including virology and bacteriology, and a thorough investigative search of the flat, all of which provided negative results, each death certificate carried the single word 'Unascertained'.

REGISTRATION OF THE DEATH

DESPITE the general rule that a death must be registered before disposal of the body, there is a relaxation of the rule in Scotland, but only as regards earth burial. Because of the transport difficulties and inclement weather in certain remote areas, delays may be experienced in getting to the registry. A body may therefore be buried, but not cremated, before registration takes place. However, the cemetery superintendent is obliged to notify the registrar if such an event occurs, so that he can await the formal registration.

THE DEATH CERTIFICATE

IN general terms, the medical certificate of the cause of death is the same throughout the UK, but there exists some important practical differences between Scotland and the other countries.

England and Wales

There is a statutory duty of the doctor who attended the deceased during the last illness to issue a death certificate *forthwith*; failing that, to see that the case is reported to the coroner. This is done by information being passed to him personally, or to request the registrar to do so, as part of his duties. Usually a personal contact with the coroner is the quicker procedure.

The problem arises if the attending doctor is away from the practice at the time of the death of his patient, for no other doctor may legally issue the certificate, even if he is aware of the facts of the case. Hence a large number of cases are reported each year to the coroner.

The English certificate requires the certifying doctor to state if and when he has seen the body after death. If he has not, but some other doctor has, then this is indicated on the certificate. Not that failure to do so will invalidate the certificate, providing that the certifying doctor has seen the now deceased during the last 14 days of his life, but there are many cases and situations in which it would be prudent to view the body. There can be no premature issue of a death certificate.

Attached to the death certificate there is a 'Notice to informant'. The certifying doctor is required also to complete it, and send it off also *forthwith*. As this supplement is required by the registrar before the death can be registered, it is customary to hand it, together with certificate, to the person who is responsible for going to register the death.

Scotland

There is a greater laxity pertaining to the issue of the death certificate as compared to the English procedure.

First, there is no requirement upon the doctor who issues the certificate to have been in attendance on the deceased during the last illness. Any registered doctor who has sufficient knowledge of the medical facts of the case is lawfully eligible to do so. In practice many death certificates are issued by police surgeons and forensic pathologists who do so under the legal proviso that they have made a just and reasonable enquiry and issue them 'to the best of his knowledge and belief'.

Second, there is nothing on the certificate to indicate when the deceased was last seen alive, unlike the English certificate.

Third, there is no space on the form to indicate to the registrar that the doctor has notified the case to the procurator-fiscal, such notification being done on a purely informal basis.

Fourth, there is no supplement 'Notice to informant' on the Scottish certificate.

Lastly, there is no need to issue the certificate '*forthwith*'. The medical practitioner is required to issue it at any time within seven days of the death. Even then no penalty is incurred for delay unless, after a request from the registrar, he omits to do so within a further three days. It is under this arrangement, that a body may be buried before the registration of the death has taken place.

Northern Ireland

The procedure differs from that in England and Wales in a few details. The age of the deceased is not required, nor whether the death has been followed by a post mortem examination. The length of the 'last illness' during which the doctor was in attendance is extended from 14 days to 28 days. The death certificate must be delivered to the registrar for the district in which the person died, or was ordinarily resident immediately before death, within five days. There is no 'Notice to informant' to be issued, and there is no indication as to whether the coroner has been informed.

THE INFORMANT

THE list of persons eligible to act as informants is similar throughout the various British legal systems.

It includes persons present at the death, any relatives of the deceased, the deceased's executor, the occupier of the premises in which the death occurred, any person who found the body or who has charge of the body and will dispose of it. The latter will include the police and the local authority social work department. The duties of the person involved are in addition to those which include reporting the death to the coroner or the procurator-fiscal.

The informant must attend personally at the registry and provide additional information, if possible. After registration the registrar will then issue a certificate for disposal and this is then handed to the funeral undertakers.

DISPOSAL BY EARTH BURIAL

PROVIDED that the death has been registered and the informant has received a certificate for disposal from the registrar, then disposal by earth burial may take place. The formalities are completed by the return to the registrar of a certificate of disposal by the funeral undertakers. There is no general statute stating how, when and where a body is to be disposed of; only the laws of public health which in general terms govern the method of disposal. Usually a body is buried in a specially appointed place, but there is no law prohibiting burial elsewhere, providing permission from the land owner has been obtained and that the public health laws are observed.

DISPOSAL BY BURIAL AT SEA

APART from expediency in times of war, it is unusual for a body to be disposed of in the deep waters around our coasts. This is perhaps surprising, considering that Britain is a maritime nation with a great sea-going tradition.

The regulations are similar to those for an earth burial, namely: registration of the death and the receipt of a certificate for disposal. The local port authority or harbour master is notified of the request through the funeral director, who, together, arrange for a vessel to sail beyond the three miles national boundary and then to deposit the coffin into deep waters. The coffin is prepared by the inclusion of a quantity of old iron or other heavy ballast and the drilling of a series of holes in the base and sides to allow the sea water to enter.

Once the coffin has been 'committed to the deep', it is virtually impossible to recover for further examination, unlike an earth burial.

A possible unforeseen problem is the relative ease by which a secret homicide could remain undetected. One way to prevent such a happening would be for the registrar to insist on the same strict rules which are enforced in the case of disposal by cremation to be applied to each sea burial.

DISPOSAL FOR MEDICAL RESEARCH

MANY people each year discuss with a variety of professional people the desirability, or otherwise, of leaving their bodies to be used 'for medical research'. This is the usual form of words used to represent an

103

anatomical dissection at a university medical school. On the other hand, where express directions have been left for certain organs to be removed 'for transplantation purposes', then effect is given to these specific instructions and the remainder of the body is disposed of in the usual manner, by burial or cremation.

Before the body can be removed to the anatomy department, there must be a valid death certificate followed by registration and a statutory delay of 48 hours after death. All the personal details are forwarded to the Inspector of Anatomy – usually the Professor of Anatomy. No dissection of the body can take place; nor indeed can any organ be removed, if there is any objection from the nearest known relative, despite what the now deceased himself requested.

The body remains must finally be disposed of within two years, either by burial or cremation.

DISPOSAL BY CREMATION

CREMATION is the ultimate method of disposal, reducing the body to a few pounds of a gritty, grey ash. By the same token it is the ultimate method of preserving a secret homicide. It is impossible to detect any drug or poison in the ash because the extremely high temperature generated in the cremator volatilizes almost all the biological and chemical substances of the body. Only elements such as calcium, magnesium and phosphorus remain in the ash.

It follows, therefore, that extreme caution must be exercised by all concerned to exclude any suspicion of criminality or medical negligence before the body is destroyed.

The safeguards are embodied in the Cremation Acts 1902 and 1952, and the Cremation (Scotland) Regulations 1935, 1967 and 1985. In practice they are set out in a series of documents which must be completed to the satisfaction of the medical referee, an overseeing official appointed under the Cremation Acts. He is a medical officer nominated by the crematorium and appointed by the Home Secretary or the Secretary of State.

The first step is the issue of a medical certificate of the cause of death and the registration of the death as set out above. Then follows a somewhat complex procedure.

Form A

This is an application form to cremate the body. It contains a series of questions to which the applicant (a member of the family, an executor, a trustee etc.) must give full answers. In summary, it asks whether the deceased left any specific written instructions as to the disposal of his remains, in particular, any opposition to cremation. The applicant must also state whether there is any reason to suspect that death was due directly or indirectly to violence, poison, privation or neglect. The application must be countersigned by a responsible person who knows the applicant.

Form B

The form is a lengthy questionnaire and must be completed by the medical practitioner who was in attendance during the last illness. The doctor must answer all the questions and he must see and identify the body after death, even if it means an inconvenience by reason of place or distance involved. If he is a relative of the deceased, or if he has any knowledge of any pecuniary interest in the death of the deceased, he must disclose it. He must state the cause of death and declare that he has no reason to believe that death was due to violence, poison, privation or neglect, or that there are any reasons or unusual circumstances such as would require a public inquiry. He then signs the form, on soul and conscience, as being a true statement.

Form C

This is a confirmatory medical certificate in which a second registered medical practitioner confirms the views, opinions and answers expressed by the first doctor in Form B. The doctor who is eligible to complete Form C must have been registered for not less than five years, must not be a relative of the deceased, nor a relative or partner of the doctor who completed Form B, and he must examine the body and have made personal inquiry before completing the document. He must be satisfied as to cause of death and state it, declaring also that he has no reason to suspect anything unusual or unnatural in the death.

Recently, a change in the procedure may supersede the need for Form C. If the deceased died in hospital or an approved institution and an autopsy was made by a registered doctor of not less than five years' standing and the findings of the autopsy form the basis of the cause of death as stated on Form B, then there is no necessity for Form C.

The three forms A, B and C are then submitted to the medical referee at least one full working day before the day of cremation. If the forms are in order then the final document is issued.

Form F

This is the final document completed by the medical referee, and is the authority to cremate, provided that he is satisfied that all the requirements of the Cremation Acts have been complied with and there exists no reason for any further inquiry.

When the superintendent of the crematorium receives Form F he can proceed to cremate the remains.

Form G

After the cremation, the fact that it has taken place, together with a summary of all the details leading up to the cremation, are included in this form which is retained at the office of the cremation authority.

Other forms which are used, albeit less frequently are the following.

Form D

The medical referee has statutory powers to order, or even carry out himself, a post mortem dissection before he authorizes cremation. This he will do, if there if any irregularity or discrepancy in the Forms A, B and C. It is usually asked for when there is some minor medical problem which requires clarification or rectification. If there is a gross error or omission it is more than likely that he will report the matter to the procurator-fiscal or coroner, who then will institute further proceedings.

If the medical referee does invoke his discretionary powers, the findings of the pathologist are reported to the referee by means of Form D.

Form E

When a death has been reported to the procurator-fiscal or the coroner, because of the suspected unusual circumstances surrounding the death, a medico-legal post mortem examination will take place. This will be followed by a legal inquiry according to the different statutory rules in Scotland and England, in order to ascertain the precise cause of death. If the relatives then wish the body to be cremated, Form E is issued in both jurisdictions permitting the cremation and replaces Forms B and C. It allows the medical referee to proceed and furnish Form F.

Form H (for England, Wales and Scotland)

Mention was made above of the procedure for the disposal of a body for medical research. If the remains are to be cremated at the end of the two years, Form H, completed by the Professor of Anatomy, or the head of the department, is sent to the medical referee in order that he can authorize the cremation.

Form H (Northern Ireland)

The form is an application for the cremation of a still-born child, made wherever practicable by the father or mother. The form is then made a solemn declaration before a Justice of the Peace or a Commissioner for Oaths. The form is then forwarded to the registered medical attendant or certified midwife.

Form I (Northern Ireland)

This is the certificate of the registered medical attendant or of the certified midwife, if no doctor was present at the still-birth or has examined the body. An attestation that the child was still-born and that there is no reason for reporting the still-birth to the coroner, completes the form.

Both Forms H and I are then sent to the medical referee to await his authority to cremate.

DISPOSAL OF STILL-BIRTHS

A STILL-BIRTH must be registered, by means of a special Certificate of Still-birth, before it is lawful to dispose of the body. A still-birth is defined as: 'a child which has issued forth from its mother after the 28th week of pregnancy, and which did not, at any time after being completely expelled from its mother, breathe or show other signs of life'.

The definition of still-birth in Northern Ireland is

the same as above, but it includes the phrase 'or extracted' after 'completely expelled'. Therefore the statutory definition makes specific provision for delivery by Caesarian section, as well as by natural delivery.

The certifier may be either a registered medical practitioner or a certified midwife, by reasons either of having been in attendance at the birth or, if absent at the birth, having subsequently examined the body of the child.

There is provision on the Still-birth Certificate for a declaration that the child was still-born, before any medical aid was available and that the facts were communicated to the certifier. A possible difficulty may arise here, that the certificate is issued on the word of a lay person, perhaps the mother herself. It might be prudent in this case for the doctor or midwife to consider requesting an autopsy before committing their professional opinion to the certificate, to obviate any later suspicion of an unnatural cause of death.

A still-birth must be buried or cremated. There can be no donation for medical research.

DISPOSAL OF FOETUSES

A FOETUS expelled dead from the mother before the 28th week of pregnancy does not come under the law in the same way as does a still-birth (after 28 weeks). Viability, in legal terms, does not begin until after the 28th week; therefore in the case of the foetus dead before 28 weeks, there is no legal requirement for registration, and the disposal therefore is done with decency and discretion and within the bounds of the

Public Health Acts.

A recent recurring problem concerns the foetus that is born, or is delivered alive before 28 weeks' gestation and then dies also before 28 weeks. Such a situation may arise due largely to the advanced technology of maintaining foetuses alive in an endeavour to allow the mother to have her anticipated child. Whilst as a matter of fact the procedures of birth and death have taken place, albeit before the legal age of viability, it would be accurate in medical terms and ethically correct for the parents, to issue certificates of birth and death, with a covering note to the registrar for his consideration as to the form of registration and subsequent statistical considerations.

5   SUDDEN AND UNEXPECTED NATURAL DEATH

ALTHOUGH from the description given above a 'natural' death has no obvious criminal or accidental causation, it nevertheless becomes of some concern to the forensic pathologist simply because of the difficulty, or even impossibility, on the part of the family doctor in being able to furnish a certifiable cause of death. He believes the person died from natural causes, but is unsure as to which one.

Many a patient, having suffered for a long time from a serious chronic disease, is suddenly and unexpectedly discovered dead. The practitioner is then in a dilemma as to whether or not to issue a death certificate. He is unsure as to the precise cause of death. Was it caused by some unsuspected intervening agent, an abnormal development of the existing chronic disease, or even a new disease altogether?

It is because of the unexpectedness of the death, and the fact that he cannot entirely exclude any vestige of suspicion, that the doctor must notify the coroner or the procurator-fiscal of the unusual circumstances.

The numerous causes of sudden natural death may conveniently be classified according to the different anatomical systems of the body.

CARDIOVASCULAR SYSTEM

DEATHS resulting from diseases and disorders of the circulatory system account for the vast majority of sudden natural deaths. They are considered under diseases of the vessels, the heart muscles and the heart valves. In some cases there is an overlap from one system to another.

Ischaemic heart disease

The interruption or interference with the blood flow to the heart along the coronary arteries will have profound effects on the heart itself. In the extreme, it will cause the heart to suddenly cease functioning; in less extreme cases, areas of the heart will fail which in turn causes a chain reaction and finally the complete failure of the heart. Ischaemic heart disease, or the insufficient supply of blood to the heart muscle, is the most important single factor in causing sudden natural death. In Glasgow and the West of Scotland are found not only the highest incidence of coronary artery disease in the whole of Europe, but also the largest number of deaths from this cause. Regrettably, the causes still remain largely unknown.

At autopsy, one or more of the main branches of the two coronary arteries may show a severe disease process. There will be a deposition of soft white or yellow necrotic fatty material on the lining of the

113

arteries. Sometimes it is uniformly laid down, but more often it is very irregular in appearance. This material, known as atheroma, reduces the lumen of the vessels and this interferes with the blood flow. Over the years the deposits of the atheroma become infiltrated by calcium, converting the areas of 'soft silt' into brittle, hard plaques. These very severely obstruct the vessels, and their presence encourages the formation of a blood clot which completely occludes the 'pin-hole' lumen and prevents further blood flow.

In about 30 per cent of cases a complete occlusion by a recently formed thrombus can be found, depending on the care taken on examining all the diseased vessels. Sometimes the vessel is completely blocked by atheroma having been displaced from the lining of the artery. Often a piece of plaque is partially dislodged and acts like a flap or valve, thereby obstructing the blood flow.

Probably the most frequently seen pathological entity is generalized severe narrowing of all the main vessels, so that when extra demands are made on the heart, as in excitement, stressful situations or a demand for extra muscular activity, the heart attempts to meet the need but fails through an insufficient blood supply to itself. This is termed cardiac insufficiency and may result in partial heart failure or total failure. The term ischaemic heart disease embraces all these aspects of coronary artery disease.

One term which is extensively used by doctors to describe a cardiac death is that of *myocardial infarction*. It is used rather too loosely by medical and nursing staff alike. It is a true pathological entity and not a clinical state. It is better to use the term ischaemic heart disease, or coronary artery disease in general discussion of a case.

When a coronary vessel becomes suddenly block-ed by atheroma or a blood clot, the interference to the flood flow results in a rapid degeneration or even death of that part of the heart muscle which depends on that particular blocked vessel for its blood supply. The process of muscle death causes intense chest pain and alerts the patient and the doctor to what is hap-pening. The affected part of the heart muscle is de-scribed as having become infarcted, and the process is described as myocardial infarction.

After a recent coronary occlusion, the areas of the infarcted muscle will depend on how major the vessel was in terms of how much muscle it supplies; and the efficiency of the nearby surrounding network of blood vessels, the collateral circulation, to assist the affected area. When death occurs very shortly after the coronary blockage, the infarcted area may not be recognized on naked-eye examination. It requires at least 24 hours following the occlusion and before death occurs for the pathologist to be able to disting-uish areas of dead muscle from the unaffected heart muscle.

Fortunately not all myocardial infarctions will re-sult in sudden death. Many a patient will give a his-tory of having had a series of 'heart attacks' from which he has made a reasonable recovery. The pa-tient may recover, but the affected area of heart mus-cle cannot do so. The dead muscle is removed by biological processes and firm fibrous scar tissue is laid down in its place. But scar tissue is not contractile like muscle and it weakens, stretches, and becomes thin. Given sufficient time the thinned area dilates and bulges outwards to form an *aneurysm*, or localized swelling. This may then rupture leading to death.

115

A further complication of a myocardial infarction is a sudden, often silent rupture of the heart, whilst the soft dead muscle is still in place and before any reparation can begin. Rupture of the heart by either means results in a large intra-pericardial haemorrhage. The presence of so much blood in a confined space presses on the heart and interferes with the normal contraction and expansion, thereby leading to sudden death. Such a catastrophe usually occurs several days after the original myocardial infarction.

Hypertensive heart disease

An enlargement of the left ventricle of the heart with accompanying increase in the thickness of the muscle wall will result in a raised blood pressure, frequently to a level twice as high as normal. This is often seen in adults of later years. Such an enlargement is often not accompanied by a strengthening or supporting of the blood vessels in the body, so that rupture of vessels is frequently seen in the presence of hypertension – raised blood pressure. One common example is the rupture of a cerebral artery. This is discussed more fully below.

The cardiac enlargement is almost always limited to the left ventricle, the three remaining chambers being usually within normal size. In many cases the cause for the enlargement is unknown, when the term *primary* or *essential hypertension* is used. Equally the enlargement may occur without appreciable symptoms, although as the hypertrophy progresses the patient requires treatment for the effects of the raised blood pressure. Death occurs quite suddenly and unexpectedly. There may be an incident of exertion, anger, emotion or stress but equally the death may follow a period of rest.

One reason for the sudden collapse and death is that the mass of heart muscle has 'outstripped' its own blood supply, so that when called upon to exert a greater effort to meet a stressful situation, the coronary arteries, which frequently are healthy and fully patent, have not become secondarily enlarged and are simply unable to supply the extra blood to meet the demand. In effect, it is similar to the situation in ischaemic heart disease. If, in addition, there is also coronary atherosclerosis present, the combination of a decreased vascular supply and an increased muscle mass leads to ischaemia and sudden death on the least exertion, or even no exertion.

When both conditions are present, the death certificate should record both pathological entities

Aortic valve disease

The condition is usually confined to males over the age of 60. It is a primary degenerative disease limited to the cusps of one heart valve, i.e. the aortic valve. It is not related to the other valvular diseases such as rheumatic heart disease or bacterial endocarditis. It is found more frequently when the aortic valve has a congenital defect such as two cusps, instead of three, although the degree of distortion, calcification and destruction of all the valve cusps sometimes makes it difficult to know exactly how many cusps existed.

Sudden death results because of the failure of the hypertrophied left ventricle to force the blood through the diseased and narrowed valve. An alternative reason is that the disease process may spread out from the valve and impede the entry of blood into the ostia of the nearby coronary arteries.

Cardiomyopathy

The word means pathological processes affecting the heart muscle, without specifying anything in particular. It is a 'rag-bag' into which a host of differing pathological conditions are put together to explain some cases of sudden cardiac death. Some examples are: chronic alcohol use, foci of bacterial and viral infections, degenerative states such as amyloidosis and enlargements of the heart of unknown origin. Usually the sudden deaths are to be found in otherwise healthy young adults.

Ruptured aortic aneurysm

This is a common cause of sudden death in late middle-aged or elderly patients. The most common variety is a large bulbous swelling in the abdominal aorta. The swelling may be to one side or anteriorly or even uniformly spread around the wall. They usually arise as an atheromatous degeneration of the aortic wall just below the origin of the renal arteries and may be limited to the aorta or they continue downwards to the bifurcation and even beyond to involve one or both common iliac arteries. The aneurysm can become very large, filled with old, non-organizing blood clot, and yet present with no symptoms until the wall becomes so thin that it bursts, causing a massive retro-peritoneal haemorrhage.

A variant of this degenerative condition is termed

a *dissecting aneurysm* of the aorta, and unlike the atheromatous variant is found most frequently in the thoracic aorta, predominantly in the first part of the aorta and involving the arch. The rupture occurs within the media, the middle of the three layers of the aortic wall. A split occurs in a degenerative part of the media and blood quickly breaks through the inner, intimal layer and enters the newly formed space. The pressure of the blood then extends the split further along the aorta, making a false channel. The blood may re-enter the normal lumen but usually it passes out laterally, through the outer, adventitial layer and into a body cavity. Death supervenes within a short time, but not before the patient has experienced a period of intense, searing pain, which is often misdiagnosed as that of a heart attack.

Pulmonary embolism

Many people consider this condition along with other respiratory causes of sudden death, but as the entire drama occurs within the circulatory system, it is best considered here.

It begins with thrombus formation in the deep veins of the lower legs. The veins lie in close association to the calf muscles and the bones. During a period of immobilization in bed, for example, constant pressure is applied to the muscles, thereby compressing the veins and interfering with the venous circulation. There may be an additional factor in the form of thrombo-phlebitis in the lower legs.

Other areas where venous thrombosis can occur involve the pelvic and prostatic plexuses. Pregnancy, congestive cardiac failure and obesity are common predisposing causes.

With a sudden alteration in the venous blood flow, for example, straining at defaecation, there is thrombus migration from a leg or pelvic vein. The mobile clot is now termed an embolus and is conveyed in the venous system through the right side of the heart and into the pulmonary trunk and the pulmonary arteries. The large embolus now obstructs the diminishing pulmonary arteries. This activates reflexes through the autonomic nervous system which in turn causes pulmonary artery spasm. Then follows overloading and dilatation of the right side of the heart and poor filling of the left side of the heart. The cardiac output is thereby decreased. The patient becomes unconscious and dies from impaired oxygen and carbon dioxide exchange in the lungs as well as a drop in the pressure in the cerebral vessels.

RESPIRATORY SYSTEM

DISEASES and disorders of the respiratory system are second only to the cardiovascular diseases in causing sudden and unexpected death. The main causes are massive haemorrhage in the air passages, pneumothorax, infections and asthma.

Haemorrhage in the air passages

When a massive haemorrhage occurs into the major air passages death results from an obstruction to normal respiratory gaseous exchange. In former years it was not an uncommon event but today is becoming less frequent. Erosion of a large pulmonary vessel by a malignant tumour or by an expanding pulmonary infection, e.g. tuberculosis, produces a massive bleed and death follows very shortly. In former years the frequency of syphilitic aortic aneurysms in the thorax meant that many would erode into a bronchus leading to a rapid death.

Pneumothorax

The spontaneous rupture of an emphysematous bulla on the periphery of a lung, e.g. following a bout of coughing or straining during some physical exertion, can lead to a massive escape of air into one of the pleural cavities. The vacuum normally present is lost and there is an immediate collapse of the affected lung. In the absence of special medical equipment death may rapidly ensue, especially if there is concomitant disease in the other lung or in the heart.

Infections

Whilst most chest and lung infections can produce a severe illness which may lead on slowly to death, there are a few bacterial and viral infections which can produce sudden and unexpected deaths in a very short time.

Example 1 A sports master at a large school used to spend his lunchtime break playing indoor football with some of the other teachers before returning to their classes for the afternoon. After about ten minutes of one of these sessions, the sports master said that he felt very tired and would not continue but encouraged the others to play for the remaining time. After a quarter of an hour the game finished and the members of staff went to the changing room to find the sports master dead on a bench.

Example 2 A young man, shortly to be married, was decorating his future home one evening after a day's work along with his father. The young man said that he had some tightness across his chest and that he would not continue painting. His father completed what he was doing and joined his son in another room 20 minutes later, where he found him dead.

In both these cases, as with others, there was an acute haemorrhagic bronchopneumonia. Culture and virological studies showed a florid viral infection.

Chronic bronchitis can also on occasions cause a sudden death. At autopsy many of the secondary and tertiary bronchi as well as bronchioles are plugged firmly by thick tenacious purulent secretions. The causation of the phenomenon remains unknown, but the suddenness and completeness of the plugging causes death by hypoxia.

Asthma

Sudden and unexpected deaths occur amongst asthma sufferers, even in those who have been sufferers for a long time. Asthma is the sudden and prolonged spasm of the smooth muscle in the walls of the bronchioles. As there is no cartilage in the bronchiolar wall, unlike the bronchi, to maintain the lumen open, the bronchospasm causes severe constriction of the air passages. If the bronchospasm cannot be effectively relieved by aerosol sprays and other drugs the continual constriction can lead to a hypoxial death.

In all these examples involving the respiratory system death is due to respiratory failure in the exchange of oxygen and carbon dioxide within the lungs. This may be due to obstruction in the airways, restriction in the ability to expand the lungs, allergic neuromuscular problems, and ventilation abnormalities.

CENTRAL NERVOUS SYSTEM

SUDDEN natural death related to the central nervous system is nearly always caused by haemorrhage which may occur either within the brain, or outside within the meninges.

Cerebral haemorrhage

This is often referred to as a cerebro-vascular accident, although the word accident is a misnomer. Lay persons may describe the event as a 'stroke'.

The massive bleed usually occurs either within the basal ganglia or more distally in the internal capsule. The resulting destruction, however, extends much further so that a large proportion of the relevant cerebral hemisphere is in a disintegrated state. The haemorrhage is associated with raised blood pressure, so that the victim is usually an elderly person with hypertensive heart disease and widespread arteriosclerosis, especially of the cerebral arteries. Cerebral haemorrhages may also occur in other sites such as the pons or the cerebellum but they are much less frequently seen.

Intracranial haemorrhage

The haemorrhage occurs outside the brain but within the meningeal layers. One well known cause is a sub-arachnoid haemorrhage caused by the spontaneous rupture of a small aneurysm known as a *berry aneurysm*. The aneurysm which may vary in size from 3mm up to several centimetres in diameter arises from one of the arteries at the base of the brain which together constitute the complex termed the Circle of Willis. The aneurysm is of congenital origin, which because of a muscle malformation in the artery wall, becomes gradually larger and because the wall is thin, ruptures without accompanying raised blood pressure. They may occur when the victims are sleeping as well as when they are engaged in exercise. They predominate in the young adult but when they burst in the older person there is usually some accompanying arteriosclerosis.

Example   A 23-year-old female had succeeded in her examinations. She gave a small party at her house for her close friends. She entered the room with a tray of glasses then suddenly collapsed to the floor and was declared dead on arrival at the nearby hospital. The autopsy showed a massive sub-arachnoid haemorrhage from one of three berry aneurysms.

Circulatory, non-haemorrhagic causes

The formation of a cerebral thrombus in one of the cerebral arteries at the base of the brain, or in a smaller branch within the brain may cause loss of consciousness leading to death within a short time. The thrombus is usually formed in association with a localized plaque of arteriosclerosis. A most unusual cause is that of a cerebral embolus which may arise from an area of thrombus formation within the cavity of the heart, passing upwards to the brain via one of the carotid arteries.

Epilepsy

Despite comments by lay persons to the contrary, epileptic sufferers may die during a prolonged single seizure or more usually during a series of repeated seizures termed status epilepticus. Death is due to asphyxia if the epileptic ceases to breathe or aspirates regurgitated vomit, or has an airway obstructed by the tongue.

GASTROINTESTINAL SYSTEM

HAEMORRHAGE is the main event causing sudden and unexpected death to patients who are suffering from diseases of this system. A massive bleed may occur when a gastric or duodenal ulcer erodes through the submuccosal tissues and into an artery lying close by. The profuse bleeding may pass down the intestinal tract emerging from the anus, or it may enter the stomach and be vomited up, or more frequently it will pass in both directions. The problem as to the precise cause of death arises when a person living alone and with no medical history is unexpectedly found dead at home.

Another form of dramatic fatal bleeding occurs when varicose and distended veins at the lower end of the oesophagus become eroded and burst. This usually occurs in a patient who had developed severe fatty change or even cirrhosis of the liver brought about by chronic alcohol use.

Fatty change to the liver can also produce a sudden death but the exact mechanism remains unknown. In some cases there is microscopic evidence of fat embolization to the lungs or even the heart or brain. Equally there may be a sudden disturbance to the nearby pancreas and insulin activity.

OTHER SYSTEMS

IN pregnancy sudden deaths are usually associated with haemorrhage. They are certainly infrequent but do occur when the patient is left unattended. The rupture of an extra-uterine pregnancy (ectopic pregnancy) may produce a massive intra-abdominal haemorrhage which on occasions has caused death. Premature separation of a placenta praevia may both cause severe exsanguination unless there is medical aid. Attempts at abortion by inexpert persons may cause death either by perforation by the instrument of a major vessel, or by causing pulmonary embolus by means of air, chemical fluids or the release of amniotic fluid into the blood stream.

The adrenal gland may be related to a sudden death as a result of bilateral adrenal haemorrhage produced during a meningococcal septicaemia. Usually there is evidence of the bacterial infection elsewhere followed by adrenal collapse and death, but sometimes the discovery of the adrenal haemorrhages at autopsy is the first clue to the disease.

SUDDEN DEATH FROM UNKNOWN CAUSES

THERE is nothing more frustrating, and no case remains so memorable, than a death for which there is no demonstrable cause. All pathologists have a short list of cases where, after autopsy, toxicology, bacteriology, virology, histology, and a review of the history of the case with all the professionals concerned, there is no reasonable cause to be found. Then all the parties concerned have to content themselves with accepting the situation that the cause of death is unknown.

One very special group of deaths which still remains a mystery is the sudden death in infancy syndrome, but this will be discussed elsewhere (Chapter 12).

Other categories include reflex cardiac deaths during or following minor surgical or medical procedures, the strange deaths of apparently fit and healthy young persons during some sport or game, and on a worldwide scale the deaths of healthy persons who have been cursed to die. These deaths invite further research into their causation.

6 WOUNDS AND INJURIES

WHILST it is the sole responsibility of the medical practitioner to express a firm opinion as to the nature of a wound or an injury, it is nevertheless in the wider interests of a case under investigation that police officers and other professional persons should learn to acquaint themselves with the various medical words used during a clinical or a post mortem examination. In other words, both medical and non-medical attendants should be able to discuss together any relevant medical findings. This can be quite fruitful, because each will bring to the discussion ideas, facts and suggestions from different standpoints.

THE DISTINCTION BETWEEN A WOUND AND AN INJURY

THE two terms, unfortunately, are frequently used interchangeably, the one being substituted for the other, even when referring to the same lesion. It probably does not matter too much which word is used during the initial examination and discussion, but when it is a matter of writing and discussing reports, then it is far better that the correct word be used.

There is no statutory definition of either a wound or an injury. However, the courts have decided, at least in England, that to constitute a wound there must be a surface breach which passes through the entire thickness of the skin, or a mucous membrane, into the underlying tissues. This means, in effect, that mere scratches and surface grazes are not wounds; neither are deep-seated lesions such as bruises, ruptured muscles or tendons, nor even fractures. They are described as injuries. The difference between injuries and wounds is therefore one of anatomical description and therefore relatively unimportant to the outcome of the case, as in practice charges of serious assault, or assault endangering life, will cover the entire range of the findings.

For the purpose of the rest of the chapter, the word 'injury' will be used in a general sense to encompass all the different types, whilst the word 'wound' will only be used in its specific context.

SOME FUNDAMENTAL RULES FOR EXAMINING INJURIES

Note carefully all the injuries

A common mistake that is easily made is to overlook small lesions. It is so easy to find oneself staring at a gaping wound, or becoming fascinated at the sheer savagery of an attack, that smaller, less prominent wounds seem to pale into insignificance. Now it is quite understandable to act like that at first, but the important rule is that all injuries must be noted. The converse is also true; the whole body should be fully examined in order to discover injuries, even in sites where they are least expected.

Record all the findings

Once the body has been fully inspected and all the injuries located, their presence must then be documented. The doctor will, of course, make his own record, but it can also be useful to an investigating officer to make his own personal record.

There is no single scheme which can be recommended in preference to any other. It is very much a personal choice. Some doctors use printed protocols consisting of a series of anatomical diagrams on which sketches of the injuries can be made. Others prefer to use a printed check-list of all the anatomical sites, on which ticks or comments can be added. A third method is to describe in detail each injury, noting its site with reference to fixed anatomical landmarks. For example, a stab wound on the front of the chest can be described with reference to the mid-line, the nipple-line and the clavicle. There are occasions when a number of injuries are so close to each other that they can best be understood by referring to the group as a whole. Simply record the overall measurements of the group.

A word of caution: make sure that the lefts and the rights are recorded accurately. Moving around a body or having the body turned over for inspection can so easily cause errors. Remember, it is the injured person's left and right that matter; not the left and right as seen by the observer.

A series of photographs by the official photographer will undoubtedly be taken, or in some cases, a video film will be made, but these cannot entirely replace the written record. Often a photograph is taken from such a close distance, and without reference marks, that it is impossible for anyone to know precisely which wound is which. At best the photograph or film is an aid to the written record.

Adopt an objective attitude to the injuries

One of the features of a medico-legal examination is that the history of the case has been relayed by several persons before the examination begins. A real danger exists that only those parts of the history which appear to have a direct bearing on the main injury are reported or firmly stressed to the doctor or the pathologist. One can so easily be influenced by what one has been told that subconsciously one is trying to marry the medical findings to the story as it was relayed. The simple rule is – try at all times to adopt an objective attitude in your work and try not to allow personal intuition or views to intrude. Often they only serve to cloud the issue.

SOME FUNDAMENTAL QUESTIONS TO BE ANSWERED

FROM the combined police and medical investigations, there are certain important questions to be answered.

How was the injury caused?

Each wound and injury must not only be carefully documented, but from the characteristics some consideration should be given as to what caused them. For example, in the case of a stab wound, was it caused by a small pocket knife or by a heavy sheath knife? In the case of a bruise, is it consistent with a fall, or was it more likely to have been caused by a kick or a punch? Sometimes it is not possible for the doctor to give an answer, nor even to hazard a guess, but from a careful assessment it is often surprising how accurate he can be. The police investigation can be greatly helped as a result of combined consultations, if some idea can be ascertained as to what instrument, if any, was used.

When was the injury caused?

There is no easy way of dating or timing an injury. It is true that there are a few specialized microscopic enzyme tests which can be employed, but the results are difficult to interpret; moreover, they are limited to the first few hours after the injury was sustained.

On the other hand, there are a number of well tried simple, rule-of-thumb methods that are generally used, such as the colour changes that occur in bruises, or the vital tissue reaction that develops around skin wounds or healing fractured bones. In spite of these characteristics, the primary question as to precisely when the injury was caused must sometimes remain unanswered.

How much force was used?

During the examination of an injury, the question is always posed: what degree of force was used? Just as with the problem of timing or dating an injury, precise figures or calculations are unavailable. Much depends on the area of the striking object. Was the same degree of force concentrated on a small area such as with a hammer-head, or over a large area, for example with the use of a flat piece of wood? The two resulting injuries will be markedly different although the same measure of force was used. One must also take into account the amount of resistance offered by the damaged tissues. Was the blow taken up by fatty springy tissues, such as the abdominal wall or by a hard bony area such as the head?

The answers to these questions just cannot be expressed in mathematical terms. The best that can be achieved is to limit the answer to the use of four possibilities: a small degree, a moderate degree, a considerable degree, or a severe degree of force. Naturally this raises the question as to what is meant by these terms, for it is a personal, very subjective matter. Nevertheless, their use in medical reports, without trying to define them, does provide sufficient flexibility to account for minor individual differences and as such, they can be useful, so long as everybody realizes that these descriptions are only approximations.

Has the injury contributed to death?

In the case where multiple injuries are present, it is very important to indicate, where possible, the injury or injuries which caused death as distinct from those which are merely incidental and non-life-threatening. Usually it is obvious, but not always, and so it highlights once again the need to note carefully all the injuries which are present.

The most commonly seen injuries can be classified as follows:

1 Abrasions
2 Contusions
3 Lacerations
4 Incised wounds
5 Defence injuries
6 Penetrating wounds.

Other injuries possessing more specialized features, for example those injuries associated with firearms, explosions, electrical accidents and road traffic accidents are considered elsewhere.

ABRASIONS

UNDER this heading come scratches, grazes, impressions, pressure or friction marks. An abrasion occurs when the surface layers of the skin are damaged. It may result from a frictional movement between the skin and a roughened surface, or to simple, firm, downward pressure on the skin. An abrasion can be said not to be a wound at all, but a superficial injury, because the damage inflicted does not extend through the full skin thickness and into the underlying tissues. Nevertheless an abrasion is of great investigative importance and has certain characteristics.

It is present at the precise point of impact

This seems quite obvious, but it does emphasize the fact that definite, firm contact was made at a particular site. If a number of abrasions are found on various parts of the body, consideration must be then be given as to when they were inflicted – all at the same time, or over a period of time.

It may exhibit a definite pattern

A pressure abrasion sometimes retains the clear imprint of the causative object. The tread of a motor car tyre, the ply of a piece of electrical flex, the stippled design of a knitted garment; are all examples of a pattern left on the skin which has contributed to the understanding of the case.

It may show a certain direction

When a roughened surface makes sliding contact with the skin it will produce a series of thin, linear parallel abrasions, at one end of which there may be a number of very small curled skin tags at the point where the sliding ceased. The effect is similar to the curled shavings produced when wood is planed (see Figure 6.1). These two features may help to determine the direction of the injury. It is worth remembering that when a moving object slides on a stationary person, the direction of the object is *towards* the skin tags, but when a moving person slides against a fixed object, then the direction of the body will be *away* from the skin tags.

135

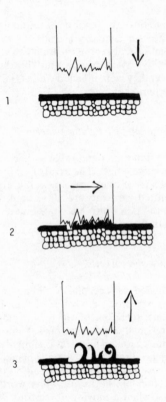

FIGURE 6.1   MECHANISM OF ABRASION

Example A cyclist was struck by a following car one dark night, on a left-hand bend of a country road. The boy received fatal head injuries and the driver was charged with causing death by dangerous driving. The motorist claimed not to have seen the cyclist until just before impact. He blamed the bend in the road and also that there was no rear red light on the cycle, but police examination of the lamp showed it to be battery operated and fully functional.

The conflict of interests was resolved by a study of a series of minor abrasions on the right side of his face. The direction, by lines and skin tags, was clearly identified as passing from the ear to the nose.

One reasonable explanation was that the boy was standing by his cycle leaning over the back wheel, perhaps adjusting the chain, thereby obliterating the rear light which was fixed just below the saddle. The right side of his face was a presenting part to the oncoming car which, as part of the head injuries, grazed the right side of his face from his ear to his nose. The court accepted this explanation.

Directional abrasions are sometimes found, not on the victim, but on the assailant, as a defensive action by the victim. In a sexual attack, parallel linear abrasions may be seen on the man's face, arms or back, caused by the woman's fingernails. Establishing the direction of the abrasions might be of evidential value in corroborating the woman's account of the incident. In addition, microscopical and serological examinations of the fingernail scrapings, in these circumstances, may provide additional evidence.

It may suggest severe internal injury

A relatively trivial abrasion may be the only indication of a more serious underlying lesion. If the abrasion is ignored, the consequences may be embarrassing, if not serious.

> *Example* The site of an abdominal abrasion on a young child who had fallen from his small tricycle was not appreciated by the family doctor. His failure to appreciate that the abrasion indicated the precise point of impact and that the force was transmitted to the internal organs, was the reason that the doctor failed to diagnose a ruptured spleen, which nearly cost the child his life.

Ante mortem versus post mortem abrasions

We have seen that an abrasion is the result of pressure applied to the skin, but it is also important to decide whether the abrasion occurred before or after death. Before death, the continuance of a circulation of blood means that there will be a pronounced reddening of the skin in the damaged area. This phenomenon is called a 'vital reaction' and is a combined nervous and chemical response whereby the blood vessels in the area dilate and allow protein-rich fluid to pass into the affected area. Hence there is swelling and a reddening of an ante mortem abrasion.

Where skin is abraded after death, as for example in rough handling, no such vital reaction occurs, as there is no blood flowing in that area. Instead the abraded skin shows a yellow-brown, almost leathery, change to the tissues, which is known as 'parchmenting'. It is due to simple air drying of the exposed tissues.

138

CONTUSIONS (BRUISES)

A CONTUSION is caused when blunt force, applied to the skin, is sufficient to rupture the underlying small veins, with subsequent escape of blood into the surrounding loose connective tissue. The overlying skin usually remains intact or there may be an abrasion.

Bruising frequently accompanies a laceration (see below). When moderate to severe blunt force is sufficient to rupture the tissues, blood will escape into the surrounding uninjured tissues as well as through the breach in the skin. Bruising associated with a laceration may be quite extensive, spreading out far from the major wound.

The following features of a contusion are worth remembering:

It may not be present at the point of impact

A bruise may occur at any level below the skin. If a bruise is deep-seated, the blood may move along several tissue planes so that its eventual appearance just under the skin may not necessarily coincide with the point of impact. In nearly all cases there is a close relationship, but it need not be so. For example, a blow to the side of the abdomen may result in a bruise appearing towards the mid-line, because of the effect of the different muscle layers.

It may exhibit a pattern

If the blow to the skin was of a moderate force and limited in depth to the fairly firm subcutaneous tis-

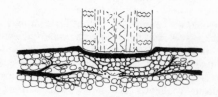

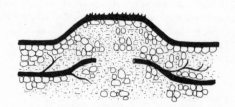

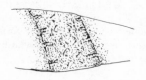

FIGURE 6.2   PATTERN OF BRUISING
CAUSED BY A VEHICLE TYRE

sues, a pattern or an outline of the object can sometimes be identified. If, in addition, there is an abrasion, the outline becomes more obvious. The outline
of the tread of a vehicle tyre (see Figure 6.2), or the
pattern on the sole of some modern shoes, the impression of individual teeth in a bite-mark, the angled
corner of a piece of furniture, are all capable of showing sufficient characteristics to be of help in identifying the causative agent.

The use of a cylindrical object, however, produces
a bruise pattern quite unlike that of any other. The
rounded nature of the object, such as a billiard cue,
broom handle, police baton or even the fingers in the
case of a severe slap, produces two parallel lines of
bruising separated by an uninjured area (see Figure
6.3). The convex shape of the object forces the blood
to the sides of the cylinder where the rapidly distended blood vessels burst.

When the deep-seated bruising occurs and if the
blood eventually finds its way to the surface there is
little, if any, resemblance to the shape of the causative object. It is just a diffuse area of altered blood,
with a blue, purple or even green colour.

It may be used as a measure of the degree of violence

Before an attempt is made to estimate the degree of
force used by looking at the size and the number of
bruises present, some consideration must first be
given to a number of physiological factors. The first
concerns the normal amount of laxity of the skin and
subcutaneous tissues. This varies markedly from
place to place. The loose tissues around the eyes, the
scrotum and the back of the hands will allow a greater

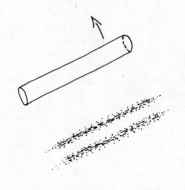

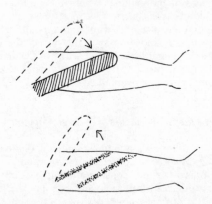

FIGURE 6.3 PATTERN OF BRUISING CAUSED BY A CYLINDRICAL OBJECT

accumulation of blood than in areas where the skin is denser or more closely adherent to the underlying tissues, such as the palms or soles, or the skin overlying the shinbones. Second, there is a wide variation throughout life in the normal distribution of fat, which helps to limit the spread of the extravasated blood. In a baby or very young child there is an abundance of subcutaneous fat and this may mask the area of bruising, giving a false impression to an otherwise serious injury. At the other extreme, in an aged person whose skin has become lax and wrinkled through degeneration of the subcutaneous tissues, bleeding from a relatively trivial blow may spread rapidly and widely, out of all proportion to the degree of force applied.

One must also be aware of the possibility of diseases or disorders of the blood which may alter the normal physiological process of blood coagulation and the repair of damaged blood vessels. Many elderly people suffer from senile purpura, in which spontaneous bruising occurs often over large areas, which because of their unusual sites, prompts the view that the person has become a victim of sustained violence.

It may be mistaken for an area of post mortem hypostasis

One of the early post mortem signs is the cessation of circulation and the pooling of blood, under the effects of gravity, in the dependent parts of the body. The colour of the skin over these areas will appear purple or a bluish-pink. However when a dependent part makes a firm contact with an underlying surface, blood cannot then enter the flattened surface blood vessels and a blanched or light pink area is seen. Therefore an inspection of the dependent part of a body will show uniformly deeply stained areas, clearly delineated from blanched, flattened areas.

If as a result of a struggle, or vigorous movements before death, the clothing of the victim becomes disturbed and rucked up, then unusual and irregular pressure points are produced on the underside of the body. The intervening spaces between the folds of the clothes will then show irregular areas of hypostasis, and after the body has been stripped, these areas may simulate bruises. Where doubt exists between a bruise and post mortem hypostasis, the pathologist will distinguish between the two by cutting into the tissues and making a naked-eye examination. If the blood is seen distributed throughout the fat and the subcutaneous tissues then it is an area of bruising, but if the blood appears to be contained within dilated blood vessels then the site is showing the normal post mortem appearance. In cases of doubt, the matter can be settled by a microscopic examination of the removed area.

Ante mortem versus post mortem bruises

The pathologist is frequently asked whether a particular bruise could have been caused after death. As the formation of a bruise depends on the flow of blood from damaged blood vessels into the surrounding tissues, and as such a flow of blood demands that there be a pumping heart, it follows that blood cannot flow out any distance after death, when clearly there is no circulation. On the other hand, because blood remains fluid for some time after death, some blood, albeit a small amount, may ooze out of a vessel, damaged after death. This could conceivably produce a small bruise, but it would undoubtedly be quite small.

In general terms, all bruises of any acceptable size are produced before death occurs.

Sites where bruising is of special interest

(i) *Neck* In cases of strangulation by ligature or in hanging, attention is always directed to the pressure site to determine the site and size of the abraded mark on the neck. Apart from the compression mark there may be no other injury and that includes bruising. If the ligature has been firmly applied and has remained without movement until after death has occurred then there may be no opportunity for the blood to escape from the compressed vessels. The absence of bruising and a vital reaction to the compressed tissues may raise the question of whether in the case of hanging a simulated suicide has been contrived.

If the ligature has been applied progressively with an opportunity for movement of the head and neck, as in a struggle, then bruising will be seen close to the ligature.

(ii) *Scapulae* Bruises are sometimes found over the lower parts of the scapulae in cases of alleged sexual assault, in which the victim has been forcibly held against the ground or against a wall. The reason for bruising and areas of tenderness at this particular site is due to the prominence of the lower part of the female scapulae as compared to that of the male. In

145

particularly thin females the bruising over these bony sites can be quite pronounced where there is little muscle or fat for protection.

(ii) *Scalp* In many cases of head injury, a bruise cannot be seen on the outside of the scalp, even in a bald head, being only visible when the scalp is reflected from the skull during the autopsy. The absence of a bruise on the outside but present on the inside of tissues is seen elsewhere, particularly in relation to flat bones, such as the pelvis, sternum and scapulae. When the affected part has been struck, the force of the blow is transmitted through the tissues causing damage to the innermost vessels as they are compressed against the hard underlying bone. Thus the haemorrhage is internal rather than external.

(iv) *Sites of restraint* In the case of a person who requires to be forcibly restrained bruising may be seen as a series of small discrete circular areas, often termed 'finger-tip bruising'. These are frequently to be found on the inner aspect of the arms and forearms. Bruises can also be found close to the axillae especially when a person has been dragged along the ground on his back.

In sexual assaults, it is important to look for finger-tip bruising on the inner aspect of the thighs and around the vulva, where the assailant's hands have tried to force the legs apart.

LACERATIONS

UNDER this heading come tears, splits or ruptures of the skin. A laceration is an example of a true wound, because the entire thickness of the skin has been breached. It results from blunt force injury applied to the skin which operates in two directions at the same time. There is a downward component which crushes the skin and the underlying structures and there is a forward component which applies a stretching or shearing force to the skin. The result is an irregular shaped split through the skin and the subcutaneous tissues (see Figure 6.4).

A laceration has certain characteristics.

It usually possesses an irregular shape

A laceration is usually a ragged-edged tear with an unpredictable shape. Around the edges there is associated bruising, which is both superficial and deep to the laceration. Because of the uncertainty as to how the skin will split under the combined forces, it is rare to find a laceration whose shape corresponds to that of the causative object, unless that object has a quite unique appearance. There is an exception to what has been said. When a laceration occurs close to an underlying bone, for example the outer ends of the eyebrows, or on the front of the lower leg, it may present as a regular wound, not unlike an incised wound (see below). This may give a false impression that the wound has been caused by a sharp cutting instrument rather than by blunt force.

There may be relatively minimal bleeding

The force applied to the skin may cause the under-lying blood vessels to go into spasm; the muscle and

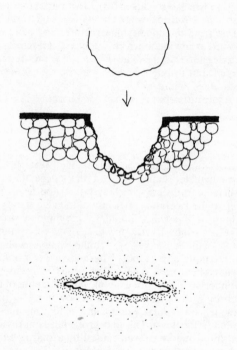

FIGURE 6.4 LACERATION BY A BLUNT
OBJECT

148

elastic layers of the small arteries contract to such an extent that there is minimal blood loss from the damaged vessels. A consequence of this phenomenon is that there is a real possibility that infection may arise within the wound. Frequently clostridial organisms and foreign debris are to be found in a lacerated skin lesion which can lead to widespread tissue destruction, requiring vigorous medical or surgical attention.

Lacerations are caused by one of three ways:

1 *When a moving object strikes a stationary victim* Thus a person may be struck by a hammer, axe, bottle etc., or he may be kicked with a heavily shod foot. In the area of accidents, falling objects, especially from a great height, can produce severe lacerations.

2 *When a moving victim strikes a stationary object* This is exemplified by a person falling down stairs, or colliding with furniture or machinery.

3 *When a moving victim strikes a moving object* A person crossing the street and is struck by a passing vehicle may receive most serious lacerations.

In all these situations the speed of the striking force and the consequent release of energy to the victim will determine the size and extent of the laceration and other tissue damage.

When lacerations are caused by kicking, there is always a considerable amount of bruising. This will be maximal in the area immediately surrounding the split skin, but it can also be seen at a greater depth and for a wider area than is the case when a punch or a blow with a weapon is the cause (see Figure 6.5).

A kick, when compared to a blow with a clenched fist, is a much slower movement. It begins slowly with the leg being drawn back behind the body, and then slowly increases its speed as the leg comes forward. The production of a kick involves the largest muscles of the body. These include the muscles of the back, the pelvis, the thigh and the lower leg. All of these combine to produce a movement of great momentum, so that when contact is made, the foot releases a large amount of kinetic energy, resulting in considerable tissue damage which includes widespread bruising around the laceration.

When kicks are delivered to the head, the site of the injuries is of some interest, because the toe of the boot or shoe usually ends up in the concavities of the head and neck. This means that the damaged tissues occur around the eyes, to the side of the nose, under the chin and behind the ear. The convex areas, namely the forehead, the point of the chin and the cheek bones usually escape injury except for minor abrasions due to the shoe sliding off these sites to end up in the hollow places.

INCISED WOUNDS

UNDER this heading come cuts, slashes or slicing of the skin thus the expression 'an incised wound' must be used with care. When the word 'incised' is used, it implies that the skin has been cut or damaged by means of a sharp-edged instrument. This may be a knife, a razor, or even a sharp piece of glass or metal. An incised wound must be distinguished from a stab wound (see below), although it must be admitted that

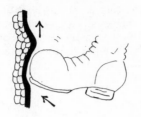

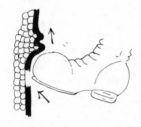

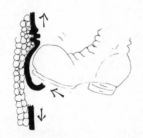

FIGURE 6.5   LACERATION CAUSED BY KICKING.

Note the splitting of skin by overstretching with production of typical 'flap'

on occasions elements of both types of wounds can be found together in the same skin lesion.

The seriousness of an incised wound depends on both the site of injury and the depth to which the cut has been made.

An incised wound has the following characteristics.

The length of the wound is greater than its depth

Some incised wounds, especially those caused on the face, may be very long, and appear quite serious; yet in depth they only just penetrate the tissues under the skin. They are usually inflicted for the purpose of disfigurement and to cause pain rather than to kill the victim.

When reporting the presence of an incised wound, there is often a fascination to know the number of sutures which the surgeon has inserted. It is of far more value to know the length of the wound and its site than a stitch number. In treating an incised wound of the face, the surgeon is aiming at a good cosmetic result. He wants to produce a hairline scar, and to do that he inserts a large number of closely placed sutures, to prevent any gaping of the wound along its length. The number of sutures is therefore meaningless, and usually he never counts them! Sometimes a surgeon may use only one suture, which is a long continuous sub-cuticular suture, where the suture disappears under the skin at one end of the incision and reappears at the other end. The reporting of one single suture to treat the incision therefore is meaningless.

WOUNDS AND INJURIES

The incised wound is like a surgical incision

Just as the surgeon produces a clean, straight-edged cut through the skin, using the minimum of downward force, so too is the normal incised wound made. The direction of the latter may wobble and deviate from the straight line, but there is no raggedness in its appearance. Moreover there is no associated bruising around its edges. The wound is not necessarily deep, although its depth may vary throughout its length, unless there is a clear homicidal or suicidal intention to extend downwards to cut the larger deep-lying blood vessels.

There is profuse haemorrhage

Because there is only a small amount of downward force involved when an incised wound is made, there is an insufficient pressure applied to the cut arteries and arterioles to cause them to go into spasm and restrict the blood flow. Therefore an incised wound will readily bleed profusely and, unless some external pressure is applied, the unrestricted flow of blood will result in serious blood loss. Usually superficial incised wounds will stop bleeding after a while by natural means, but it is unwise to assume that that will happen in every case.

Sometimes a small, relatively insignificant superficial wound, for example on the inner aspect of the wrist or in the groin, may prove fatal, because a major artery, lying just under the skin, has been transected.

There is little opportunity for infection

An incised wound is rarely an infected wound. Because the amount of bleeding from an incision an be excessive, the possibility of infection within the wound is remote. It is therefore good practice to allow a reasonable flow of blood before treatment, to assist in the removal of bacteria and other foreign material from the wound.

One special form of an incised wound, which is particularly life-threatening, is that found on the front or side of the neck. This is therefore generally referred to as a 'cut-throat' wound.

Cut-throat wounds can be described as: suicidal; homicidal; or accidental, that being the order in which they are most frequently seen.

Suicidal cut-throat wound

The number of suicidal wounds far exceeds the other two forms, being fairly high on the list of causes of suicide.

The characteristics of the wound are as follows:

(i) *The site on the neck* This largely depends on whether the person is right- or left-handed. The wound is usually found on the opposite side of the neck to the hand which held the cutting instrument.

(ii) *The appearance of the wound* It is an obliquely downwards directed wound, beginning usually below the angle of the lower jaw and ending close to or at the mid-line of the neck. It may be a deeply produced wound from the start, although it is more frequently seen as a shallow wound at the commencement, becoming much deeper as it approaches the mid-line.

(iii) *'Hesitation' or 'tentative' marks*   A very important feature, and one which virtually clinches the diagnosis, is the presence of 'hesitation' or 'tentative' marks alongside or quite close to the main incision. They are always present. In fact, one would not like to diagnose the wound as being suicidal in their absence. They demonstrate the mental anguish and disturbed thinking of the victim who was trying to discover whether the incision would be painful, and whether it would produce a large release of blood, escaping blood being seen as life running away. Whatever the reason, it serves to help establish the cause of death (see Figure 6.6).

(iv) *Jugular vein and trachea*   The wound will usually open the jugular vein and often the trachea, but it is surprising how often the carotid artery is spared because of its protected position so close to the large sternomastoid muscle.

(v) *Other features*   There may also be tentative marks at the wrist as well as on the neck (see Figure 6.6). These may be trivial, but they are important, being part of the depressed mental state, and should be looked for.

The deceased may have left a suicide note and this should be enquired after.

The deceased may have made previous attempts to commit suicide by other means. Enquiries in this direction should not be overlooked.

The uncommon, but highly important, condition

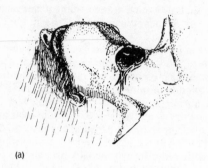

(a)

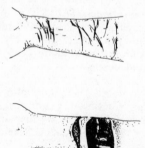

(b)

FIGURE 6.6 (a) SUICIDAL CUT-THROAT (b) SELF-INFLICTED INCISED WOUNDS OF THE WRIST

of cadaveric spasm (see chapter on changes after death) may be present. The knife or razor may still be present in his hand.

Death usually results from profuse haemorrhage or from the presence of air in the heart. This was drawn in through partly opened veins in the neck. A large quantity of air in the right ventricle prevents the heart from normal functions.

Homicidal cut-throat wound

The main points of difference from the suicidal wound are the following:

(i) *Single wound*   There is usually a single wound, which is deep along its entire length. There is frequently some bruising in the walls of the wound, due to the forceful downwards pressure used in making the wound.

(ii) *Site on neck*   The wound usually occurs lower down on the neck. It is more horizontally placed and is found more to the front of the neck than on the side.

(iii) *There will be no hesitation marks.*

(iv) *Abrasions and bruising*   There may be abrasions and bruising under the chin and on the upper part of the neck. These are caused by the resistance of the victim, struggling against a hand or an arm which was forcing the head backwards.

(v) *Torture marks*   Rarely, but important to identify, there may be long thin superficial incisions, slightly deeper than abrasions, lying irregularly around the neck. These have been termed 'torture marks', inflicted to terrorize the victim before the fatal blow. There should be no difficulty in distinguishing them from suicidal hesitation marks.

Accidental cut-throat wound

This occurs infrequently, but when it does there is usually a good background report and sufficient circumstantial evidence to support the diagnosis. The wound, or wounds, may be caused by flying glass, such as follows an explosion, or the victim may have fallen through a glass door or a plate-glass window, whereby he cuts himself on the jagged edges.

The injuries are irregular in shape and may occur anywhere on the neck, in a manner unlikely to have been caused by anybody intent on inflicting injury on the neck.

DEFENCE INJURIES (PROTECTIVE INJURIES)

A defence injury may be found on that part of the body which has been instinctively raised, or put out in front, to prevent an anticipated blow from causing damage to some other, more vulnerable, part of the body.

When present, it is believed that the victim saw the blow coming towards him, in the form of a sharp-edged instrument, or an object capable of inflicting blunt force injury, and in an act of self-defence he received incised wounds, stab wounds, bruises or other less serious injuries to his forearm, hand or wrist. They may also be found on the thigh, though these are less frequently seen.

Throughout the upper levels of the animal kingdom there are two basic instincts. The first is to protect the eyes. The theory expounded is that a blinded animal inevitably becomes a dead animal, as it cannot see to feed itself, and no other animal will assist it. The second basic instinct is to protect the organs of procreation for the continuance of the species, namely the external genitalia.

Any blow delivered to the region of the head and upper trunk causes the head to be turned away and the arms to be raised to ward off the attack. If a knife has been used, then incised wounds or stab wounds may be found on the outer aspect of the wrist and forearm. The discovery of incised wounds on the palm of the hand and in the flexures between the joints of the fingers indicate an intention to grasp the knife to prevent injury elsewhere.

If a blow is aimed at the groin or lower trunk, the body responds by bending forward and raising a leg so that the external genital organs are protected. Defence injuries may be found on the lateral aspect of the raised thigh or knee, or even the backs of the hands.

Defence injuries are important to a police investigation because their presence may lend support to the view that a blow received by the victim elsewhere on his body was probably not accidentally caused, but was intentional.

PENETRATING WOUNDS

UNDER this heading come stab wounds and perforating wounds. A penetrating wound results from forceful contact with a pointed firm instrument. A common example is the wound which results from a thrust or a lunge with a knife (see Figure 6.7). The weapon need not necessarily be sharply pointed, but if it is not, then a greater degree of force will be needed to penetrate the skin. In practice, the most frequently encountered instrument to produce a penetrating wound is a sharp-edged, sharply pointed knife, so much so, that the term 'stab wound' is almost synonymous with a knife wound. This is regrettable, because it tends to exclude from one's mind the use of any other instrument. A farmer's pitch-fork, a carpenter's tool, a steel knitting needle or a piece of engineering equipment can all produce fatal penetrating wounds, but will be overlooked, if the term 'stab wound' is reserved only for a knife wound.

Whilst a single stab wound may have been caused intentionally, the possibility must never be overlooked that the wound could have resulted from an accident or, more rarely, from an act of suicide.

One of the great imponderables in forensic medicine is that of distinguishing a wound caused by a positive thrust by an assailant, from the accidently produced wound caused by the victim rushing his armed assailant and impaling himself on to the knife.

The chief characteristics of a stab wound are as follows.

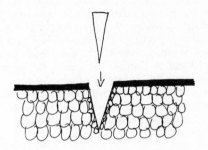

FIGURE 6.7   STAB WOUND

The depth of the wound is greater than its length

This contrasts with the incised wound, where the length of the wound was greater than its depth. Sometimes, however, there may be a combination of both wounds, so that care must be exercised to see whether there is penetration of the body to a sufficient depth to warrant the use of the term 'stab wound' instead of a 'deep incision'.

The size of the wound will bear no relationship to its depth. Small stiletto-type knives can penetrate to a great depth whilst producing a surface wound of only a short length.

It results in internal injury

Unless one has seen the body organs displayed and removed at an autopsy, it may come as a surprise just how close to the surface of the body some of our vital organs lie, and because of this fact a stab wound, on passing through the skin and subcutaneous tissues, may very quickly and easily penetrate the heart, lungs, aorta, the liver or some part of the alimentary tract. These organs are so well supplied by blood that any damage to them will probably be life-threatening.

One of the casualties resulting from the re-shaping of the present-day school curriculum is the subject of human biology, for which only a small amount of time is allowed. As a result many young people of average intelligence are remarkably ignorant of the general structure and function of their own bodies. This is repeatedly highlighted with the death of a youth following a street brawl or a gang fight, when the young accused person strenuously asserts that he had no idea of the presence of the vital organs so close to the skin. He intended to draw blood and inflict pain but was shocked to learn the full extent of his action.

The length of the wound relates to the width of the weapon

Once a stab wound has been made, the presence of elastic fibres in the connective tissue around the hole will cause the wound to gape open, thereby converting a slit-like entry wound into an oval shape. The true length of the wound can only be measured once the two edges have been brought together. The measurement will therefore be the width of some part of the knife blade. Where that point on the blade is will be related to the depth of the wound. Many knife blades alter their shape and width as one examines them from the sharp point to the hilt or the insertion in the handle. If a suspect knife is available for measurement the length of the wound when applied to the blade may help in estimating the depth of the wound. A blade whose width at any given point is wider than the wound clearly cannot have caused the wound, because it could not have gone into the skin. However, when the width of the blade is less than the length of the wound, then two deductions may be drawn. Either it is the wrong knife because the blade is too narrow, or it may be the right knife because on entry or on withdrawal, or both actions, a rocking action was caused, whereby the angle of entry and the angle of withdrawal are different. The result of this abnormal movement is to create a skin wound greater in length than the horizontal width of the blade. Thus a small knife can make a large wound.

The shape of the wound may represent the shape of the blade

A double-edged weapon will usually produce a symmetrical pattern with sharp angles at each end of the skin wound. On the other hand, a single-edged knife with a thick back to the blade, such as a butcher's knife or a heavy sheath knife, will cause one sharp end to the wound and a blunt, or 'fish-tail' appearance to the other end.

A knife with a serrated edge, for example, some kitchen knives or a blade with a knick along its length will produce a ragged appearance to one end of the wound. These will be seen best by means of a hand lens.

It is often difficult to state with certainty the depth of a wound. The organs of the chest and abdomen are mobile and when the body is examined in the horizontal position, they may occupy a position different to that when the body is upright. This means that when a stab wound has ended in an organ such as the lung or the intestine the pathologist will have to estimate the probable depth rather than give a precise depth.

It must also be remembered that the fat under the skin can be easily compressed so that when the knife is forcibly pushed into the abdomen, the anterior abdominal wall with its layer of fat can be pressed back towards the vertebral column by the hilt or the handle of the knife. This compression will allow the tip of the blade to go even further into the body. Thus when the blade has been withdrawn and the abdominal wall has returned to its normal position, the depth of the wound is considerably greater than the blade length.

To assess the degree of force required to make a stab wound several factors must be remembered. The force depends largely on:

(a)   the shape of the blade, and whether single- or double-edged;

(b)   the sharpness of the blade, and whether single- or double-edged;

(c)   the degree of protection afforded by any clothing or body coverings;

(d)   thè particular organs that have been penetrated, such as bone or other hard tissues;

(e)   whether the knife has ended its journey in soft or hard tissues;

(f)   any movements on the part of the victim which might 'trap' the knife, causing it to bend the blade or even break it.

A knife that has penetrated 'up to the hilt' often causes some bruising around the edges of the wound, or at the sharp ends of the wound, and this bruising will increase with the force with which the hilt strikes the skin.

It is not possible to measure the force required to make a particular stab wound, but taking all the above-mentioned factors into acount the best that can be achieved is to use a descriptive term such as light, moderate, considerable or severe force, and leave it at that.

SUMMARY

THERE is a causation for all the injuries on the body; they do not happen by themselves, therefore give considerable attention and thought to what is displayed. Some may be fresh injuries; others may be older and in the process of healing, but each must be thought about. Do not overlook the small and apparently insignificant marks, simply because a large obvious wound is staring you in the face.

Make note of everything; you cannot have a second opportunity once the body is away.

Finally, before reaching a firm conclusion, make certain that all the alternatives have been adequately discussed and considered.

7 HEAD INJURIES

Of all the wounds and injuries caused by blunt force or sharp instruments, those affecting the head fall into a special, important category, because of the secondary involvement of the brain and nervous system. Head injuries account for about 25 per cent of all deaths due to violence and about 60 per cent of all fatal road accidents. Furthermore head injuries form one of the most difficult areas of diagnosis in accident and emergency medicine, with strong medico-legal overtones, including possible claims for negligence.

For all professional workers dealing with a victim of a head injury, one of the most important considerations is whether there is, or has been evidence of unconsciousness. No matter how short the period, the fact, or even the possibility of it having occurred, is sufficient reason for the victim to be kept under close observation for at least a day, to exclude the slow development of an intracranial haemorrhage. It is good practice for any professional person handling an unconscious patient to assume the presence of a head injury until it is shown to be due to some other cause. It is not wise to assume the semiconscious state of an intoxicated man found lying in the street to be due solely to alcohol; there may well be an associated head injury. This is especially important when it involves a person conveyed to a police station for overnight detention. His very quiet state may be the only outward sign of a head injury, received during a fall whilst drunk.

In this regard, the victim must be transferred to hospital to be under medical supervision, and for the necessary diagnostic tests to be carried out to detect a possible skull fracture, cerebral haemorrhage or brain swelling due to oedema.

THE FUNDAMENTALS OF A HEAD INJURY

THE application of force to the head, either directly, e.g. a blow to the head by a heavy object, or indirectly, e.g. on falling backwards and striking the head on the ground, may result in a single injury or a combination of injuries. A single injury may be seen on the scalp, whilst a combined injury can involve the scalp, the skull, the meninges and the brain, depending on the nature, and the degree of force applied to the head.

The scalp

Injuries to the scalp can include abrasions, contusions, incised wounds and lacerations and these have been discussed elsewhere (Chapter 6). However the tissues of the scalp are remarkably dense with the blood vessels lying mainly on the inner aspect of the scalp, close to the skull. When direct force is applied to the scalp, which is closely adherent to the underlying rigid skull, the softer scalp tissues are crushed. This may result in a deep-seated bruise on the inner aspect of the scalp, which may not be visible on the hairy outer aspect, even when the head has been shaved. But if the force is more severe, a full-thickness laceration is produced which may be irregular in shape, and can often reproduce the shape of the striking object. Frequently the laceration is also seen as a straight linear tear. Because the scalp is well supplied with blood vessels on its inner aspect, full-thickness lacerations usually produce profuse to serious haemorrhage.

The skull

With increased force applied to the head, the skull will fracture, a term which simply means a break or disruption of bone. This may occur anywhere on the vault or across the base of the skull, the latter being much more serious. The term 'simple fracture' is used when the scalp overlying it remains intact, and 'compound or open fracture' when there is an open route from the fracture site to the outside air, either by a deficiency in the scalp over the fracture, or by jagged ends of bone protruding through the scalp.

The term 'simple fracture' can be misleading because under the intact scalp the bone may be broken into several pieces (comminuted) or a piece may be separated and embedded into the surface of the brain (depressed) quite apart from a straight linear break in the bone.

If the fracture is linear, with no depression of the bone edges, the fracture may not be of any great

169

importance in so far as it affects cerebral function. If, however, the line of the fracture crosses an artery on the surface of the bone, the resultant tearing of the vessel can produce a dramatic intracranial haemorrhage. When present over the occipital region, especially if the line of the fracture is vertical, a linear fracture can be diagnostic. The probable cause is that of a man falling backwards and striking his head on the ground.

The depressed fracture, mentioned above, occurs when the striking face of an object, such as a hammer, separates a piece of bone from the vault, the piece often having the same shape as the causative weapon, and forces the bone fragment, or a free edge of bone, inwards and on to the brain. Such an event will cause localized brain damage with tissue swelling, haemorrhage and some brain dysfunction.

Blunt force injury to the skull may also result in stellate fractures of the vault with a localized area of injury and several linear fractures radiating out widely from the central point, usually following lines of least resistance through less dense bony areas.

In children and young adults there may not be a fracture through one of the skull bones itself, but rather the blunt force may cause partial separation of some of the bones along the tortuous suture lines. Suture lines are the interdigitating borders of two adjacent bones which enable one bone to 'knit' with its neighbour. This separation is usually accompanied with local bleeding and is described as a 'sprung-suture' or the springing apart of the sutured borders of the bones.

The skull is not of uniform texture or solidity, but rather is made up of two compact layers, known as tables, separated by bone of a loose texture. On occasions a blow of only moderate force may produce a fracture in one table and not in the other. Such fractures may be missed on a radiological examination of the skull, being only apparent at the autopsy.

One unusual, but clearly recognizable, fracture may be found in the base of the skull. It presents as a ring around the foramen magnum, although the fracture line may not necessarily lie very close to the foramen. It is caused by the transmission of a force along the vertebral column to the base of the skull, driving the central part of the base up towards the brain. It occurs when a person falls heavily on his feet or on his buttocks. Rarely, a ring fracture may be found when a force is applied downwards on to the top of the head, but then the 'ring' is usually incomplete.

INTRACRANIAL HAEMORRHAGE

BLEEDING inside the skull, which is usually but not always, caused by blunt force injury to the head, may be divided up into the following (see Figure 7.1):

1 Extradural haemorrhage
2 Subdural haemorrhage
3 Subarachnoid haemorrhage
4 Intracerebral haemorrhage

Extradural haemorrhage

Extradural haemorrhage is almost always associated with a skull fracture, usually involving the temporal bone. If the fracture line crosses one of the branches of the middle meningeal artery which is closely

FORENSIC MEDICINE

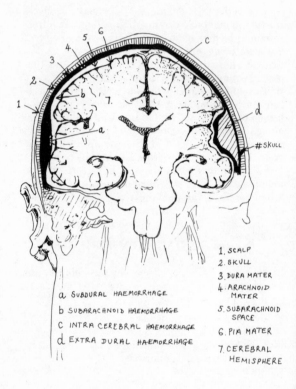

a SUBDURAL HAEMORRHAGE
b SUBARACHNOID HAEMORRHAGE
c INTRA CEREBRAL HAEMORRHAGE
d EXTRA DURAL HAEMORRHAGE

1. SCALP
2. SKULL
3. DURA MATER
4. ARACHNOID MATER
5. SUBARACHNOID SPACE
6. PIA MATER
7. CEREBRAL HEMISPHERE

SKULL

FIGURE 7.1   SAGITTAL SECTION OF HEAD AND INTRACRANIAL HAEMORRHAGES

172

applied to the inner table of the temporal bone, the artery may be torn, resulting in brisk bleeding. The accumulating blood slowly forces the very firm dura mater membrane away from the skull, enlarging the space occupied by the blood. The dura is slowly pushed inwards, compressing the brain.

The clinical picture is important and must be recognized because this form of intracranial haemorrhage if diagnosed early enough is amenable to surgery and the patient's life can be saved.

Immediately after the blow to the side of the head, there is usually a short period of concussion (a 'knock-out' blow), following which he regains full consciousness with a normal behavioural pattern though perhaps complaining of a severe localized headache. This state, described as the 'lucid interval', will last from many minutes up to many hours, after which there is a noticeable change in his demeanour. The longer the lucid period, the more likely it is that the victim will be somewhat vague about the initial injury if, indeed, he remembers it at all.

Blood continues to accumulate in the extradural space producing severe headache, and leading inexorably to confusion, stupor, coma and finally to death. As the bleeding is very limited in its site, the blood thickness produces decisive local pressure on the underlying brain. If diagnosed early enough treatment is directed to the evacuation of the local collection of blood thereby reducing the pressure on the brain, and sealing off the site of the bleeding.

A common cause of failure to diagnose this important form of intracranial haemorrhage is the frequent association of the head injury and acute alcohol intoxication. A man is seen to fall whilst drunk and is removed into police custody because he is drunk and incapable. His arrest may take place during the lucid interval following his heavy fall and probably he is noisy, obstreperous and even violent, giving the typical appearances of a 'weekend drunk'. During his stay in police custody he quietens down, giving the impression of 'sleeping off his drink'. His quietness may be simply because he is resting but equally it may be misdiagnosed as he passes into coma and then dies. A death in police custody automatically calls for an inquiry. The need for close observation is therefore obvious. One way of ensuring that he is not becoming comatose is for the observer to be made aware of the possibility of a head injury and to physically awaken the man and turn him on to his other side every 15 minutes. If any deterioration is suspected, he must be admitted to hospital.

Subdural haemorrhage

Whilst extradural haemorrhage was invariably due to trauma, what can be said of subdural haemorrhage is that it usually is due to trauma of considerable force. On the contrary sometimes the injury is not remembered by the patient, or considered to be of no consequence, despite some superficial abrasion or bruise being present. Rarely this form of haemorrhage may not be related at all to trauma, the bleeding occurring as a result of some blood clotting disorder or to chronic alcoholism. On close questioning, however, there may have been some former traumatic incident, but so trivial as to be of no concern to the normal person. Subdural haemorrhage occurs from the rupture of the veins or a large venous sinus lying in the space between the dura mater and the arachnoid membrane.

When the subdural haemorrhage is in association with a serious head injury there is only a short period of lucidity, if at all, as the bleeding is produced fairly quickly and immediately causes an increased pressure on the brain with rapid loss of consciousness. As the bleeding is usually on one side or the other of the brain, the effect of the pressure presents a flattening of the surface of the brain on the side opposite to the haemorrhage. If the patient lives long enough the brain is 'pushed' across the cranial cavity and pressed directly against the dura by the ever-expanding blood clot on the other side of the brain.

Not all subdural haemorrhages are necessarily fatal. Some never even compress the brain. They may produce no more than mild to moderate pressure symptoms and these may be evacuated surgically, but this is exceptional.

There is one form of subdural haemorrhage which is frequently seen in children and old people and it is usually of a chronic nature. Bleeding from small cortical veins on the surface of the brain is usually the cause, which then become walled-off and altered in character over succeeding years. They may not produce any clinical signs at all.

Subarachnoid haemorrhage

Haemorrhage occurring in the sub arachnoid space, that is the space between the arachnoid membrane and the very thin pia mater which envelopes the brain, may occur in three ways.

(i) *Natural disease* It is fairly common to discover subarachnoid haemorrhage occurring in the absence of any trauma or unnatural stress to the head. It arises from a spontaneous rupture of an aneurysm arising from one of the basal arteries of the brain which constitute the Circle of Willis. The cause is readily confirmed at autopsy, when on occasion more than one aneurysmal dilatation may be seen. Most are believed to be of congenital origin, there being some structural deficiency in the musculature of the artery concerned. They are usually fatal, but some leaking aneurysms may be surgically treated.

(ii) *Complication of a head injury*   If the blow to the head is capable of producing a subdural haemorrhage by the tearing of some cerebral veins, then the degree of force is usually sufficient to tear other veins passing across the subarachnoid space and causing marked haemorrhagic staining to the cerebro-spinal fluid within the subarachnoid space.

(iii) *Injury to the vertebral arteries*   In recent years a particular form of subarachnoid haemorrhage has been recognized, whereby a collection of blood is found at the base of the brain and around the upper part of the brain stem, and in the absence of any conventional head injury. It is now attributed to a traumatic rupture of one of the vertebral arteries, or one of its branches, in the region of the first cervical vertebra. Rarely the rupture may be in the basilar artery, formed by the junction of the two vertebral arteries.

There is always a history of a localized blow to the side of the neck, usually just below the ear. The external injury may be quite trivial, but on dissection of the layers of muscle and soft tissue down to the lateral process of the first cervical vertebra, bruising is usually seen in several places between the layers. Rarely there is a fracture of the cervical process but if not then there is always bleeding into the tissues along the top of the process and up to the base of the skull.

It is believed that the blow stretches and then tears the vertebral vessel at some point along its tortuous route from the vertebra into the cranial cavity. There is very brisk bleeding which gathers around the upper part of the spinal cord and compresses the vital centres necessary for the maintenance of life.

Alcohol intoxication plays a significant part in many cases, in that the reflex response of the neck muscles endeavouring to counter the blow is largely lost. Death is usually very rapid but on occasions it has been reported as being delayed for up to an hour or more.

Intracerebral haemorrhage

This may be described in two forms, the distinction depending to a large extent on whether the blunt force injury is to a stationary head (an active force) or whether the head is moving when it receives the blow (a passive force).

When a stationary head is struck, the resulting damage to the scalp, the skull, the blood vessels in association with the meninges and the brain is all localized to the one area. The intracerebral component usually consists of contusions of the superficial area of the brain immediately under the blow with, perhaps, some extension of the bruising into the deeper areas beneath. One describes this local brain damage as a 'coup' injury, and is readily understood in terms of the whole pattern of injury.

When however a moving head hits a hard surface, such as the ground (though the scalp and skull damage are found to be lying at the precise point of impact), the damage to the brain is usually diametrically opposite to the point of impact. Thus if an intoxicated man falls on to the back of his head then extensive contusions of the brain are to be found not on the occipital area, but on the undersurface of the frontal poles and also involving the temporal poles with extensions of the bleeding deep into the underlying brain tissue. The main point is that there is no significant damage to the occipital region, i.e. underneath the fracture line.

This well recognized injury is known as a 'contre-coup' brain injury. It all depends on the moving skull coming to an abrupt halt slightly quicker than the brain contained within it. The brain, as it stops, becomes 'squashed' momentarily at the impact site thereby 'pulling loose' from the blood vessels at the front of the head. The vessels become stretched and tear the surface of the front of the brain giving rise to haemorrhage and brain damage.

The significance of the finding of a contre-coup injury is that it indicates a movement of the head at the time that the blow was received.

As well as superficial haemorrhages, deep-seated intracerebral haemorrhages are often seen, particularly in the corpus callosum. This part of the brain acts as a connecting bridge between the two cerebral hemispheres. Haemorrhages are found here when there has been severe rotational or shearing movement of the brain, such as can be found in road traffic accidents where there is a severe deceleration force affecting the entire head.

Deep-seated intracerebral haemorrhage may be

quite unconnected with injury. It is a common finding in a sudden and unexpected natural death. It is referred to as a 'stroke' and results from spontaneous rupture of diseased arteries within the brain usually associated with raised blood pressure.

BRAIN SWELLING

FROM time to time following blunt force injury to the head, the victim progresses fairly quickly into deepening coma and dies without any perceived localizing signs of damage apart from perhaps some superficial abrasions. This fatal condition is termed cerebral oedema, or brain swelling. Some neurosurgeons refer to it as 'closed head injury'. The exact mechanism remains unsure but probably as a result of a disturbance to the venous circulation an excess amount of fluid passes from the arteries into the brain substance, thereby increasing the volume of the brain. This continuing increase presses the brain against the skull, causing a generalized compression of the brain which in turn brings about unconsciousness and then death, unless surgically or medically treated.

CONCERN FOR HEAD INJURIES

THE prevention of any of these traumatic head injuries which may result in death has brought action from many varying national organizations whose concern is for increased safety. It is therefore not surprising that mining and quarrying workers, those working or visiting building sites, motor cyclists, jockeys and show jumpers and participants in many sports and games all see the necessity to wear some form of head protection. Whilst there will always be some who will argue for the ideals of individual liberty in such matters there is no denying the fact that the imposition of the wearing of hard helmets has dramatically reduced the number of head injuries which in turn has reduced the loss of life.

8 ASPHYXIA

ASPHYXIA may be defined as the result of a significant interference with the oxygenation of, and the removal of carbon dioxide from, the red blood corpuscles. Unless interrupted in some way, this interference will lead to oxygen-starvation of the brain cells resulting in death.

The mechanisms of asphyxia may be classified as follows:

1 *Mechanical*. The air passages become closed, either by internal obstruction or by external pressure.

2 *Toxic*. The oxygen–carbon dioxide exchange in the red blood corpuscles is prevented by the action on the cells of poisonous substances.

3 *Environmental*. There is insufficient oxygen in the inspired air to maintain life.

4 *Medically induced*. The flow of oxygen is interrupted, or interfered with, by some medical manoeuvre, usually in association with anaesthetic gases.

5 *Pathological*. This occurs when by reason of some disease process affecting the respiratory tract, oxygen transport to the lungs is impaired.

FORMS OF MECHANICAL ASPHYXIA

Suffocation

The term is used when the nose and mouth are obstructed. The death of an infant by suffocation always presents a problem as to its causation. It is a relatively simple matter to cause death by placing a pillow, or holding down firmly some soft material, over the face, and at the same time leaving behind no evidence of any external pressure.

If there are any signs of suffocation, and frequently there are none, then they are the general signs of oxygen deficiency. These may be venous congestion of the skin of the face, and possibly the upper part of the trunk. There are often petechial (pinpoint) haemorrhages of the conjunctivae and the eyelids as well as those appearing widely scattered in the skin of the forehead close to the hair-line.

If a hand had been used to apply continual pressure over the mouth and nose, one might expect to find small areas of finger-tip bruising on the face. Equally, there may be instead focal areas of pallor where the pressure of any object, such as the pillow, had remained in place well after death, preventing congestion from occurring in the pressure points. If an object remains in contact with the nose or mouth, pink-stained secretions and possibly vomit, may be found on the object.

The question is often asked whether a young child can suffocate itself in its sleep, by turning its head and pressing its face into the pillow. Many child psychiatrists in rejecting this idea reason that if a child experienced breathing difficulties it would naturally and reflexly move its head, so that it could breathe. On the other hand, if the child was too tightly tucked into its cot, or alternatively became entangled in the bedclothes, and was unable to move freely, it could suffocate.

In any discussion on suffocation of a child in its cot or pram, the alternative problem of the Sudden Infant Death Syndrome ('cot death') must be considered.

In former years, one form of suffocation was overlaying. It occurred when a very young child slept with its parents or with older children, and a larger person rolled over in his sleep on to the face of the baby. Some cases undoubtedly occurred when at least one of the parents was under the influence of alcohol or other drugs.

A recent form of suffocation has been highlighted with the increased use in the home of thin polythene container bags. When these are placed over the head by children, imagining themselves as spacemen, static electricity may cause a close adherence of the bag to the skin of the face making it impossible to breathe. If the adherence is sudden and panic ensues, death may occur quite quickly with only minimal characteristics of asphyxia. This is why many departmental stores supply polythene bags which contain a number of perforations.

Each year there is a small, but consistent, number of suicides in which death by suffocation is achieved by placing one or two polythene bags over the head, held in position by elastic bands around the neck.

Suffocation as a method of committing homicide in an adult is possible only where there is a great physical difference between the victim and the assailant. This may be because of relative helplessness caused by old age, ill health, or incapacity from alcohol or other drugs, or the victim must first have been rendered partially unconscious from a blow. Sometimes suffocation by this means forms part of a malicious intentional act; at other times it is seen as a misguided act to avoid a suffering patient having to undergo a supposed prolonged period of agony of pain and distress.

It is usual for the assailant to use excess force to the face, more than is necessary to kill, thereby producing bruising, abrasions or even more serious injuries to the victim.

Obstruction in the mouth

The stuffing of material into the mouth of a victim to prevent him calling for assistance is termed gagging. It is rarely done in order to cause death because nasal respiration is usually not affected. However if the material is forced to the back of the mouth it can obstruct respiration, both oral and nasal, or it may cause death by vagal stimulation resulting in a reflex cardiac arrest. It is not unknown for a mentally handicapped person to commit suicide by stuffing large amounts of newspaper into his mouth as far back as the pharynx thereby causing an asphyxial death.

One form of gagging is to tie a ligature across the mouth between the open jaws, so that the tongue is forced back into the pharynx to obstruct normal breathing.

I have personal experience of one fatal case where a gag was applied very firmly across the mouth. It dislodged an upper denture, which then became impacted sideways in the pharynx and larynx. In some cases of status epilepticus death has been caused by the tongue being pressed back against the posterior pharyngeal wall, occluding the airway.

An uncommon form of asphyxia occurs when the weight of the body, or some external pressure, produces a very forcible flexion of the head and neck on to the chest, thus obstructing the normal air flow in the larynx and pharynx.

Obstruction in the larynx

The impaction of a foreign body, either between the vocal cords or immediately above them, is termed choking. Even a very small object such as a fragment of food or a small amount of fluid can cause distressful coughing and serious breathing difficulty until it is dislodged, but when a large bolus of food is impacted in the larynx, there is a marked stimulation of the vagus nerves, which almost always results in sudden death.

This catastrophe is frequently seen in association with alcohol intoxication or with mental disease, especially if the victim is also edentulous, and where there is a disregard for careful chewing and swallowing of food.

Babies and young children are at risk because at such an age they have the habit of putting all small objects into their mouths with the danger of choking and probable death. Occasionally adolescents and young adults, who have used chewing-gum whilst participating in some physical sport, have accidentally choked on it and would certainly have died but for the prompt action by colleagues in dislodging it.

Obstruction in the lower respiratory tract

This may occur in several forms. First, a small object, such as a haricot bean, an inhaled piece of dental equipment or tooth, or a nut or bolt held in the mouth during a piece of work, can obstruct the entrance to one of the bronchi or one of the major branches. This may cause death by vagal stimulation or, at a later date, bring about a local infection leading to bron-chopneumonia and a lung abcess. Second, obstruc-tion may follow inhalation of regurgitated vomitus. This sequence of events is often a problem for the pathologist. Did the inhalation of the vomit cause an asphyxial death, or did death from some other cause, as part of the dying process, bring about the inhala-tion of vomit?

There is no doubt that in many cases of head in-jury, or an acute intoxication either by alcohol or respiratory-depressant drugs, the cough reflex – the ability to clear a partially obstructed larynx and pharynx – is depressed or totally suppressed. When this occurs there is no natural defence mechanism to prevent an obstruction of the lower air passages which leads to an asphyxial death. On the other hand, a person dying from a hypoxial death, for example carbon monoxide poisoning, hepato-renal failure or acute coronary insufficiency, may inhale vomitus as an agonal or terminal event.

Hanging

Hanging, or death by suspension, is caused by con-striction of the neck by a ligature in such a manner that the weight of the body, or a part of the body, is pulling against the ligature. It is this feature of the weight of the body acting against the ligature that distinguishes hanging from ligature strangulation. The distinction is more than academic; hanging presumes a suicide, but ligature strangulation presumes homicide.

In hanging, the suicidal nature is nearly always apparent from the circumstances, such as the point of suspension, the use of a ready-to-hand ligature, the choice of location – usually one which is private, well-known, and where the victim will not be found in time to interrupt his plans – and sometimes a 'suicide note'. Homicidal hanging, and suspension of a victim of murder to look like suicide, are very rare.

Accidental hangings can be divided into two distinct categories.

(i) *Sexual asphyxia*   This phenomenon is predominantly engaged in by young males, although on occasions middle-aged men or rarely an elderly man may become involved. It is rarely, if ever, associated with females. The most important point to remember is that one is not dealing with a suicidal hanging.

The principle believed in is that by partially asphyxiating himself, the boy or young man will increase his sexual fantasy or awareness, and also prolong orgasm during masturbation.

Usually the victim protects the skin of the neck by placing a towel or a garment under the rope. He may also add to his masochism by tying himself in ropes, but leaving his hands free to release the rope around the neck and also to reach the genitalia. There may be pornographic literature close at hand.

The safety margin between partial hypoxia and total anoxia is dangerously small, so that it is believed that death supervenes before the victim is aware of the danger, and if aware, it is too late to do anything about it. The partial suspension may be accompanied by, or occasionally replaced by a plastic bag over the head, and possibly augmented by the insertion into the bag of butane or propane from camping gas containers.

An inspection of the beam in the attic or garden shed across which the rope had been fixed, will frequently show a series of small indentations, consistent with former, successful, episodes.

(ii) *Non-sexual cases* Most cases of non-sexual accidental hanging involve children, who play with swings, ropes, ladders, or get their head trapped between fixed bars. The circumstances are usually readily understandable to support a diagnosis of accidental death, but dealing with small children entangled in clothes, the bars of the cot, or a restraining harness may require extra thought to exclude homicide.

(iii) *The characteristics of hanging* The ligature in hanging will usually be something close at hand, that does not require too much preparation. In the house it is usually a length of clothes line or window cord; more recently a television co-axial cable or a length of plastic-covered electrical flex. In places of confinement, such as a prison cell, torn strips of sheet or pillow linen, boot laces or a trouser belt have been used.

The ligature mark on the neck is usually a groove which is deepest opposite the position of the knot. The knot may be on the left or right side of the neck, or at the occiput; suspension by a knot sited below the chin is rare. When the ligature is arranged using a fixed knot, the groove is horizontal on the side away from the knot, but as the cord approaches the knot the mark on the skin turns upwards towards it, producing an inverted V. The apex of the V, where the knot is, may not mark the skin because the head tends to fall away from the knot.

A slip knot or running knot quickly tightens around the neck when the body weight acts against it. The rapid tightening tends to produce a mark on the neck which is more horizontal than V-shaped, and the knot itself becomes embedded in the skin.

It does not require the full weight of the body to successfully accomplish hanging; the weight of the upper part is quite sufficient. Hanging can be effected from a low point of suspension. A victim may sit on the floor and use the door handle to fix the ligature and then let the body fall away from the sitting position. This tends to produce a horizontal mark around the neck at about the level of the upper border of the larynx. The horizontal appearance, as opposed to the inverted V form, closely resembles the mark of ligature strangulation.

The main post mortem findings are those of congestion of the tissues above the ligature with petechial haemorrhages, but only if the carotid arteries have not been completely occluded. If the pressure is sufficient, by reason of the weight of the body against a rapidly tightening rope, there may be no difference to the skin above or below the ligature. If the body has remained suspended for a few hours, post mortem lividity, with numerous large petechial haemorrhages, will be seen in the forearms and the lower legs.

Under the ligature the skin may appear white with congested borders, but more frequently, because of the movement of the ligature during tightening, the skin will be abraded, later turning brown and parchmented, a drying, post mortem change.

Examination of the internal structures of the neck frequently shows surprisingly little, if anything of note. Fracture of the hyoid bone and/or the thyroid cartilage is rarely seen and probably the only consistent finding is superficial bruising on the surface of the middle region of one or both sterno-mastoid muscles.

The causation of death in hanging is the sudden, rapid closure of the large vessels – the carotid arteries – and possibly the vertebrals, and the external jugular veins on each side of the neck. This results in immediate obstruction to the cerebral circulation. There is rapid unconsciousness and death must follow in 5 to 10 minutes.

Ligature strangulation

Asphyxia by ligature strangulation is caused by applying a ligature to the neck in such a way that the pressure is exerted solely by the ligature. The weight of the body plays no part in the constriction, and thus ligature strangulation is distinguished from hanging.

Most victims of ligature strangulation are women and not infrequently there is also an associated sexual assault. The instrument used is anything likely to be close at hand. These include stockings or tights, scarf, belt, cord, telephone or electrical flex. There may be several turns around the neck, although frequently there is only one, fastened firmly at the back by a knot.

The marks seen on the neck will correspond to the turns of the ligature, but also there may be abrasions and bruising produced during the struggle by the fingernails and hands of both the assailant and victim as well as the ligature. There may be a clear imprint of the pattern of the ligature. In a recent case the ridges of the nylon border of a cardigan matched perfectly the series of parallel abrasions on the front of the neck.

Occasionally within the ligature there may be found some object such as a stick or spoon, to twist and tighten it, acting like a tourniquet.

At post mortem examination the mark may be in the form of a groove, or more frequently it will show a series of bruises and small abrasions running horizontally partly, or rarely completely, around the middle portion of the neck. Multiple turns may produce a complex bruised pattern which can best be understood when the ligature is still in place.

Internally the main feature of note is the presence of widespread bruising. The bruising is seen mainly in the sterno-mastoid muscles and also in the smaller strap muscles lying on either side of the larynx. There is frequently engorgement of the soft tissues around the tonsils, the root of the tongue and the pharynx.

Whilst injury to the hyoid bone is uncommon, because the ligature is usually sited well below the bone, the thyroid cartilage is frequently fractured, especially one or both superior horns. The finding of damage to the thyroid cartilage is almost exclusively due to homicidal strangulation.

In addition there are the characteristic signs of generalized anoxia above the ligature with intense congestion, especially of the conjunctivae and numerous petechial haemorrhages. The pressure on the vagal nerves may cause rapid death before the congestive changes can manifest themselves, but usually death is slow with pressure on veins and the trachea before pressure is exerted on the carotid arteries.

One unique form of ligature strangulation involves the use of the umbilical cord to strangle a newborn baby. The problem for the pathologist turns on the question whether such an act could occur whilst the baby was still in the uterus, or during the descent of the birth canal, or after the baby was fully delivered. The problem involves the question as to whether the child was alive or dead when it finally left the mother (see Chapter 12 for a fuller discussion).

Suicidal ligature strangulation does occur but it is quite rare. It is usually seen in mentally diseased patients and then it requires a ligature made of a material which when held tight will not slip once the pull of the victim's own hands is slackened after having lost consciousness. Certain items of man-made fibre will easily slip but some woollen or cotton articles will 'grip' without any degree of slipping to effect a successful outcome.

Manual strangulation (throttling)

Death following manual strangulation is presumed to be due to homicide, it being generally accepted that suicide by this means is almost impossible, and the rare accidental causes are usually due to vagal stimulation of the heart following a playful jest, or some other essentially innocent circumstance.

The victims of manual strangulation are usually women, children or infants and frequently there are sexual overtones in each case.

In the less commonly seen cases of adult male victims, they are usually under the influence of alcohol or other drugs or have been first rendered less resistant or even unconscious before they are strangled.

Occasionally, in the case of an elderly victim, it may be carried out to end suffering from some terminal illness

Throttling is a common choice of homicide, since the agent, a pair of strong hands, is immediately to hand.

There is usually a well developed picture of asphyxia with an intense blue or purplish appearance to the face, swelling of the softer tissues such as lips or eyelids and prominent areas of petechial haemorrhages especially on or about the eyes. Frequently there is an escape of pink-stained secretions from the nose and mouth. The tongue may be protruding through the swollen lips.

The local signs in the neck region may consist of separate areas of bruising, with possible superficial abrasions on each side of the neck which may correspond roughtly with the thumbs and finger ends. If the nails of the assailant are long, then crescentic, or more frequently linear, deep scratch marks are seen. There may also be bruises in the other areas of the neck due to the victim struggling and moving the neck during the throttling process. Most assailants probably use more constraining force on the neck than is necessary to kill the victim and this is reflected by the widespread and serious nature of the internal injuries. Bruising is the most consistent pathological result and is found at all tissue levels down to the larynx and trachea. The extent of the bruising is in keeping with the breadth of the hands of the assailant and may be found over the entire front and sides of the neck, in differing degrees.

One diagnostic feature of importance is the presence of a fracture to at least one part of the laryngeal skeleton. Most frequently seen is a fracture to one or both of the superior cornua of the thyroid cartilage with haemorrhage between the broken parts spreading out into the immediate surrounding area. The higher placed and more protected hyoid bone is occasionally also fractured due to displacement by the assailant's pressure or by firm pressure on the ligament connecting the hyoid to the thyroid cartilage. If direct pressure is applied to both ends of the hyoid bone, then a double fracture will result. When this occurs, there is usually bruising within the posterior part of the tongue, because of its attachment to the hyoid bone.

It is occasionally suggested that the prominent ends of the hyoid bone and the thyroid cartilage may have been damaged by the pathologist during the dissection and removal of the structures from the neck. This proposal can be easily repudiated by the presence of haemorrhages in association with the broken parts. These can only occur during life. In any event, such a happening could only occur in careless or unskilled hands.

Other pathological findings include haemorrhage into the superficial layers of the thyroid gland and possibly the submandibular salivary glands.

Here is a good case for a block dissection of the entire neck structures after rendering the entire area 'bloodless' as described in Chapter 3. It enables discrete, small ante mortem bruises to be located and distinguished from blood-stained areas caused during the dissection when the structures are still *in situ*.

The mode of death in both forms of strangulation depends on the interaction of four mechanisms.

Some or all may also apply to other forms of compression applied to the neck. The four components are:

(i) *Obstruction to the venous return to the heart*
Stagnation in the veins implies that gradually all the available oxygen in the blood will be taken up by the brain cells with a failure to replenish the supply. The resulting anoxia will not only affect the brain tissue but will also adversely affect the state of the walls of the capillaries and other small blood vessels. There will be engorgement and over-distension of these vessels and thus, together with the detrimental effect of anoxia on the cellular component of the vessel walls, will result in multiple scattered petechial haemorrhages.

(ii) *Obstruction to the arterial blood flow* The carotid arteries in the neck form the main supply of oxygen to the brain. The vertebral arteries close to the spinal column are an important supplier of blood but to a lesser degree. A maintained manual compression of the carotids is possible but it requires considerable strength in the hands' pressure to achieve complete and sustained occlusion as compared to the application of a ligature. However, taken in conjunction with the venous occlusion, a very serious deprivation of oxygen to the brain is readily achieved.

(iii) *Stimulation of the vagal nerves* As with other forms of interference with the neck, abnormal and unexpected stimulation of one or both vagi can produce sudden death by arresting the cardiac movements. The precise mechanism is somewhat uncertain; it may be pressure on the nerves themselves, or small branches of them, or even pressure on the carotid plexus of nerves found in association with each carotid artery.

(iv) *Occlusion of the trachea* This is the least important of the four, because it is remarkably difficult by a circumferential compression of the neck to completely occlude this cartilage-strengthened airway. Nevertheless it can be done and may add the element of fear to the victim who is experiencing increasing difficulty in inspiration.

Mugging

Mention is made here of this not uncommon form of a strangle-hold strangulation, in order to distinguish it from the incorrect use of the word in vogue today, which is applied to any form of assault with robbery. Mugging should really only be used to describe the holding of the neck of the victim in the bend of the elbow. Originally it was a hold used in wrestling, but it is no longer permitted. Regretfully children at rough play hold their opponent round the neck in this manner, and occasionally serious results have been reported.

> *Example* A car owner was returning to his car at night and found several youths attempting to break and enter it. He surprised them at their work and succeeding in holding one of the youths by applying a neck-hold with one arm, whilst trying to open the car door with the other arm, in order to convey the youth to a police station and make a 'citizen's arrest'. Excess pressure applied to the neck to prevent him escaping resulted in the death of the youth.

ASPHYXIA

Traumatic or crush asphyxia

This form of asphyxia results from accidental gross
pressure on the chest, and often the whole body, by a
strong enough force to inhibit respiration by preventing the movement of the chest wall, or the diaphragm
via the abdominal wall. The external appearances of
a victim of this form of asphyxia are characteristic.
There is a deep red or blue-purple discolouration of
the skin of the upper chest, neck and head. There are
usually widespread petechial haemorrhages with
perhaps frank areas of bleeding in the eyes, nose and
possibly ears. Rarely, there is nothing to be seen externally, death having come very quickly after the
crushing incident.

The circumstances can involve a single person, for
example, a workman in a trench, when the walls suddenly collapse, or a person trapped under a load of
sand, grain or rubbish, or when part of a building falls
and traps him by the upper part of the trunk. More
dramatically, crush asphyxia can involve a crowd of
people in a situation of excitement and panic with
bodies falling on top of one another. Examples are
well known, such as the underground railway disaster
in 1943. During an air raid 173 persons were crushed
to death when someone at the front of a mass of
people hurrying down the stairs tripped and fell. A
similar disaster occurred on New Year's Day 1971 in
the Ibrox Stadium, Glasgow, at the end of a popular
football match. There was abnormal movement on
one of the stairs leading to the terraces which resulted
in 66 deaths, and a much greater number of people
injured. More recently in 1985 at the Heysel Stadium
in Brussels 39 people died when a wall collapsed during rioting. Probably the greatest recorded example

of traumatic asphyxia was in 1896 in Moscow when a mad struggle for food led to 1500 deaths.

Pressure on the chest or abdomen prevents inspirational movements to oxygenate the returning blood to the heart and lungs, and if there is additional pressure to the neck, the effects are similar to strangulation in which the venous return is impeded. Frequently one finds fractures to the ribs which compounds the difficulty in breathing. Survivors from a mass crushing experience repeatedly tell of the sensation of tremendous pressure to the body, with loss of vision, a feeling that the head would burst apart and the eyes would come out. Frequently there is urinary and faecal incontinence.

FORMS OF TOXIC ASPHYXIA

LIFE depends on an uninterrupted flow of oxygen from outside the body to the cells and tissues of all the organs by means of haemoglobin in the red blood cells. Oxygen binds itself to the haemoglobin for purposes of transport and then is released to be subsequently attached to the body cells by enzymatic processes. Toxic asphyxia implies an interruption to the transport system of oxygen. It can be by means of preventing the oxygen becoming bound to the haemoglobin or by means of disturbing the enzymes and preventing the tissues receiving the oxygen. An example of the first interruption is carbon monoxide poisoning, and for the second disturbance, cyanide poisoning.

Carbon monoxide intoxication

Carbon monoxide is a colourless, odourless gas, which is slightly lighter than air. The important property of the gas is its great readiness to attach itself to haemoglobin. In fact the affinity of haemoglobin for carbon monoxide is 300 times greater than for oxygen. The gas forms a fairly stable complex, carboxy-haemoglobin (COHb) and prevents the uptake of oxygen. The formation of COHb is cumulative so that a relatively small concentration of carbon monoxide in the inspired air can build up to produce a fatal concentration, often without the victim appreciating the danger he is in.

Carbon monoxide was readily available to the general public in the formerly used town gas supply, but with the introduction of natural gas (North Sea gas) and the widespread substitution of it for the town gas, except in Northern Ireland, the number of suicidal deaths from carbon monoxide has fallen significantly.

The ways in which people come into contact with carbon monoxide involve an incomplete combustion of a fuel source and an inefficient system of removing the 'fumes' – the products of the combustion.

Of the main sources of poisoning by carbon monoxide there are three which are frequently seen and together constitute the greatest number of deaths from this cause.

(i) *Domestic and industrial fires* Whenever a fire breaks out in a relatively confined space, with an inadequate source of oxygen to bring about complete combustion, or an inadequate escape route for the smoke and fire gases, carbon monoxide will rapidly accumulate causing death to trapped victims. This subject has been fully considered elsewhere (Chapter 10).

(ii) *Internal combustion engines* The running of a motor vehicle within a closed space, such as a garage with the doors shut, or the driving of a vehicle with a defective exhaust system can lead to a build-up of carbon monoxide within the car to the endangerment of the occupants.

A common form of suicide, now that town gas is almost unavailable, is to fix a flexible pipe to the end of the exhaust pipe in order to bring the exhaust fumes into the car. By this means the gases, which contain about 6 per cent CO, can kill a person in under 20 minutes, provided the car is sealed from within to prevent escape of the gases.

Carbon monoxide may be found in normal non-smokers, at a level from 0–4 per cent. Normal people who smoke may have levels up to 8 per cent. Very heavy smokers may reach 10 per cent. At a level of 30 per cent there is dizziness, headache, and nausea. At 40 per cent there is incoordination and stupor which passes into unconsciousness at 50 per cent. Death is inevitable between 60 and 70 per cent. The rate at which these levels of COHb are attained depends on the concentration of the gas in the inspired air together with the rate and depth of respiration.

(iii) *Inadequate ventilation* Paraffin, gas, oil-fired or solid fuel heaters depend for their comfort and efficiency on an adequate, draught-free supply of oxygen and a corresponding adequate outlet pipe or flue to carry away burned gases.

Flues blocked by rubble, birds' nests or soot are

commonly discovered during the examination of a room in which a death has occurred. Other findings include broken burners, non-regulatory replacements to fires following conversion from town gas to natural gas, and the use of items of equipment which are faulty or have been previously condemned as unsafe.

Death from carbon monoxide poisoning is therefore usually accidental or suicidal, homicidal deaths being very uncommon (despite popular crime novels). Elderly persons are particularly at risk from accidental poisoning for various reasons. There may be a strong element of forgetfulness in turning off fires or taps securely; they may be concerned about heating costs and block up every conceivable crack in the room to save the heat, thus affecting the ventilation; they may sit very close, or over, a paraffin heater which is in need of service; or they may simply use a heater in a room with an inadequate exit for the fumes.

Cyanide intoxication

Cyanide is a very good example of a poison which blocks the action of tissue enzymes, thus preventing the transfer of the oxygen to the individual cells. The most sensitive cells are in the brain, in particular those of the so-called 'vital centres', which includes the respiratory centre. The blood of the deceased remains a cherry-pink colour, because the oxygen is still bound to the haemoglobin. Two other causes for a bright pink colour must be remembered, in order that they may be excluded. One is carboxyhaemoglobin and the other is due to cold conditions, such as refrigeration of a body or hypothermia due to exposure. In the latter case death was due partly to the physiological failure of the oxygen to dissociate from the haemoglobin, this phenomenon being temperature-controlled.

Apart from its use in the biochemical laboratory, cyanide salts and gases are used in a number of industrial processes and therefore are readily available for determined suicidal victims.

There is a real danger for pathologists and mortuary room workers. First, some people are unable to smell the presence of cyanide, due to genetical reasons, and they must rely on others to tell them if it is present in the air. The second problem is that the characteristic smell of almonds, readily detected even at low levels, quickly passes off due to localized desensitization of the nerve endings in the nose and mouth, so that the worker close to the body may be unaware of the continued presence of the poison, whilst dissecting the organs. All persons involved in the investigation of a cyanide death must take extra care for their own safety.

Whilst poisoning from natural sources of cyanide, such as fruit stones, is very rare, a real problem exists in tropical Africa. The staple diet for many peoples is cassava, which when first harvested contains very high levels of cyanide in the fibrous roots. The roots must first be soaked thoroughly in water for several days, before preparations to make the flour can commence.

FORMS OF ENVIRONMENTAL ASPHYXIA

DEATHS occur simply because there is insufficient

oxygen available to sustain life. Therefore in forensic terms deaths from environmental asphyxia will be considered when the body has been removed from a situation where the renewal of air around the body has been impossible. Instances of a child being trapped in a disused trunk or refrigerator during play are not unknown. Overcrowding by a large number of persons in a confined space may lead to multiple deaths. Refugees in hiding, prisoners in transit in inhuman conditions, persons trapped in submarines, collapsed tunnels or in a collapsed building, are but a few examples of this form of asphyxial death. The physiology is such that as the oxygen concentration in the blood becomes lowered the concentration of carbon dioxide increases which in turn reflexly increases the depth and the rate of respiration, using up the oxygen more quickly. A vicious circle ensues and death follows. Whilst some purists might say that death was due to carbon dioxide, others would point to the depletion and exhaustion of the oxygen as being the cause.

Death from carbon dioxide in a concentrated form is occasionally seen and the rapidity of death indicates that it is from this gas *per se* that the person died and not from a depletion of oxygen.

Example Two cleaners were working in a ship's cabin on a luxury liner. Each cabin was fitted with an appliance in the ceiling which would release suddenly a supply of carbon dioxide to extinguish a fire. There was a delay mechanism to allow the occupants of the cabin to escape before the gas was allowed to fill the cabin. It is believed that one of the cleaners accidentally knocked the apparatus in the ceiling with her broom, and the gas poured down on them before they had time to realize what had happened, resulting in almost immediate death.

FORMS OF MEDICALLY INDUCED ASPHYXIA

MODERN forms of general anaesthesia usually involve the inhalation of a mixture of gases with a deliberate reduction in the percentage of oxygen. The control of the oxygen level rests with the anaesthetist. Very rarely a catastrophe occurs due either to human error or less likely mechanical failure with disastrous results ranging from cerebral damage to death. Such a mishap becomes a matter for a medico-legal inquiry.

FORMS OF PATHOLOGICAL ASPHYXIA

ANY pathological condition of any part of the respiratory system that results in an interference with the normal air flow to the alveoli will cause some degree of asphyxia. However, because for the most part they are well recognized medical matters and are diagnosed as such, they do not form part of the remit of the coroner or procurator-fiscal. But should death from such causes be sudden and unexpected, then naturally a medico-legal inquiry is started.

The main causes are acute laryngeal oedema; prolonged status epilepticus with spasm of the glottis and larynx; bronchitis with plugging of the smaller bronchi and bronchioles by thick, tenacious mucus; emphysema in all its forms; pulmonary fibrosis, a good example being the rapidly progressive form

seen after Paraquat poisoning; rapid growth of a neo-
plasm of the bronchus; the now less frequently seen
paralysis of the muscles of respiration by acute
poliomyelitis; and the most distressing state of death
during a prolonged acute attack of bronchial asthma.
All these examples are recognizable either by clinical, radiological or pathological examinations.

Apart from the sudden and unexpected deaths,
there is one other area of pathological asphyxia which
is of legal interest and that concerns the industrial
respiratory diseases which, by stimulating dense
fibrous and scar tissue in the lungs, can produce a
slow asphyxial death. Coal miners' dust disease,
asbestosis and silicosis are but a few of the many
industrial diseases which are likely to be investigated
for claims for compensation either by the victim or
the widow.

9 INJURIES FROM PHYSICAL AND THERMAL AGENTS AND OTHER SOURCES

THERE is a heterogenous collection of physical and thermal agents, such as explosions, electricity, cold and heat, as well as forms of medical treatment which, when used with neglect or through ignorance, can bring about disastrous results. Although they cannot be neatly catalogued, each has its own specific medico-legal importance.

HYPOTHERMIA

WHEN the loss of heat from a body is greater than the heat produced, the body becomes hypothermic. If the hypothermia is prolonged and not reversed, then circulatory failure will develop with ventricular fibrillation of the heart and death. The body has relatively good methods for protecting itself when exposed to hot surroundings, but it is very poorly equipped to adapt to cold conditions. The only mechanism for generating heat is by the most inefficient method of shivering, and this only comes into operation once the body temperature has already fallen below normal. It is a delayed response. Even then, the process of shivering slows down until it stops altogether as the body temperature continues to fall.

Hypothermia is defined as the state of a person whose central body temperature, the 'core' temperature, or high rectal temperature, is less than 35°C (normal = 37°C). When the core temperature lies between 35°C and 32°C, the hypothermia is described as moderately severe.

It is at this level that all shivering stops. However, if the person receives expert medical and nursing attention, he/she usually recovers. Severe hypothermia is defined as the state of the body when the core temperature falls below 32°C. The patient is described as being in a very grave state when the temperature falls to 30°C and recovery is usually unexpected when it reaches around 25°C.

It must be remembered by all concerned that the temperature readings are taken from high in the rectum. Any other site is useless. Also, it is useless to use a normal clinical thermometer, which does not register low temperatures. A chemical thermometer with a scale from 0°C to 100°C must always be used.

Most deaths associated with prolonged exposure to cold are accidental, slow in onset, and occur in a variety of ways. The insidious development of hypothermia emphasizes the need for all professional workers to suspect the condition in all geriatric or immobile patients during the winter months, or during unusually cold damp spells at other times of the year, who are found in a collapsed state, without a raised temperature.

Warm clothing, compatible with normal body

movements and work requirements, will afford some protection against a cold environment, but even the warmest clothing will fail to protect a person from hypothermia, at rest, when the ambient temperature is at −20°C, the working temperature of a domestic deep-freeze cabinet. For those who work in very cold climatic or industrial temperatures, electrically-heated clothing is usually required.

Apart from clothing, body fat, being a poor conductor of heat, may be of some help, in that a fat person will develop hypothermia more slowly than a thin, or purely muscular person.

The only mechanism remaining, after shivering, for a cold person to ward off the cold is for him to shift his blood volume from the periphery of the body to the central, or core sites. The effect of alcohol, so often given in the past by well-intended passers-by, serves only to dilate the peripheral blood vessels. The man has a temporary feeling of outward warmth, but the transfer of some of the blood back to the periphery from the core sites results in a worsening of the degree of hypothermia and may expedite death.

Deaths from hypothermia

The medico-legal interest in deaths from hypothermia falls into two separate areas.

The first is when death occurs in a healthy person who has been exposed to cold damp conditions. This may occur when outdoor enthusiasts, such as hill-walkers, mountaineers and people who work for long periods in the open air, are exposed to cold, wind, rain or snow. The dangers are considerably increased if, during these conditions, they are not protected by adequate clothing. It is the element of dampness that expedites hypothermia. The body can tolerate dry cold much better than wet cold, the worst situation being immersion in the cold sea, for wetness very dramatically increases heat loss.

Well known, and more appreciated by all, is the example of mild confusion and moderate hypothermia found in people drenched in a storm in an exposed place, who cannot quickly reach shelter and dry clothing.

Confusion, collapse and failure to keep moving compounds the hypothermic state which then leads to death.

The second area is when death occurs in elderly unhealthy persons, who die in conditions linked with cold, damp housing and under-nourishment. The situation is seen each winter. There are undoubtedly a number of socio-economic reasons for it, and despite much advice and help offered by the social services departments and local 'good neighbours' schemes to those at risk, deaths continue to occur from hypothermia.

Hypothermia, either incipient or real, must always be borne in mind in the lonely, house-bound geriatric person, even when more obvious diseases predominate, such as heart failure, chronic respiratory diseases and mental deterioration. It is possible that hypothermia will be the cause of death rather than the presenting disease.

Post mortem findings

On external examination, the only feature may be a bright pink colour of the skin of the dependent parts, in contrast to the normal blue/purple colour of post mortem lividity, and a brown/pink colour, usually in blotches over the skin of the face and the larger joints, such as the knees, elbows and sometimes the hips and ankles. There may be secondary findings such as superficial abrasions, if he has stumbled around in a confused state before collapsing just before death.

On occasions, especially in the open, such as on a hillside, the body may be discovered in a state of partial undress. This situation may, at first sight, suggest a sexual element in the death, especially if the victim is female. The phenomenon of partial, rarely complete, undressing, and scattering the clothing around on the ground, as part of the hypothermic state, is well known although most bizarre. It is believed to be due to abnormal stimulation to the hypothalamic region of the brain, disturbing the 'thermostat control' of the body. The brain regards the body as becoming warmer instead of colder; hence the need to discard necessary clothing.

The author has seen a number of cases where the victim before dying hides himself in strange places, under the bed, or under the floorboards, or, in one case, under a heavy wooden hat-stand in a hallway. This condition, termed the 'hide-and-die syndrome' may be the result of mental confusion brought on by hypothermia. The appearances at the scene certainly seem to be highly suspicious of homicide, until the circumstances and the autopsy findings are known.

If the pink-coloured body is found in the garage or a cold part of the house, the possibility of death from carbon monoxide intoxication must always be considered. A toxicological analysis of the blood for carboxyhaemoglobin will clarify any possible confusion with hypothermia.

An internal examination of the body may reveal very little of note, indicating that death was due to hypothermia. The gastric mucosa may show numerous, small 'punched-out' haemorrhages. Less often there are small haemorrhages in the pancreas and the upper intestinal tract, and there may be diffuse haemorrhages in the lower lobes of the lungs.

Microscopical examination frequently shows widely disseminated intravascular blood coagulation affecting the smallest blood vessels in numerous organs, including the brain.

In some elderly people, apart from frequently found heart disease and chronic pulmonary disorders, there may be some degree of poor thyroid function, in the form of myxoedema.

HYPERTHERMIA

THE ill-effects of heat, whether due to over-exposure to the sun or to the excess heat while trapped in an enclosed place, such as the boiler room in a building or the engine room of a ship, can be conveniently divided into two groups, namely heat exhaustion and heat hyperpyrexia.

Heat exhaustion

This is caused by salt deficiency and dehydration. Cases in the UK are unusual because of the relatively moderate climatic conditions which pertain as compared with the excessive daytime heat of the deserts of North Africa, the Gulf States, Western America and elsewhere.

211

The cases seen at home are sporadic and are easily explainable: soldiers on parade in heavy uniform, or participants in heavy costume in carnival parades, workers in factories, foundries or places where there is excess heat production or abnormal malfunctioning of systems designed to remove the heat produced.

Usually the symptoms can be promptly relieved by the replacement of the lost salt and water. The excess sweat produced by the heat causes excess chloride excretion, thereby reducing the blood chloride level. Other biochemical changes occur, notably a high blood urea level, and low urinary producton. The symptoms include marked, often intense, muscular cramps, vomiting, headaches and abdominal pains.

Even in severe cases, which require intravenous saline, successful results are usually quickly achieved with few if any residual symptoms.

Heat hyperpyrexia

This condition is caused by a failure of the heat-regulating mechanism in the brain. It is usually a temporary condition cured by removal to cooler conditions. The symptoms are different from those of heat exhaustion, in that there is usually no excess sweating, no cramps, abdominal pain or vomiting. The only sign is a steady rise in temperature and the victim collapses and becomes unconscious. The popular term for this condition is 'heat stroke'. One place where heat hyperpyrexia must always be considered is the operating theatre, where a patient may have to undergo a prolonged operation. The possibility can be prevented by a careful regulation of the weight of the body coverings on the patient, the humidity of the room and consideration for the prolonged exposure under the intense operating theatre lights.

Malignant hyperpyrexia is the name given to a special form of hyperpyrexia which almost always occurs under a general anaesthetic. On occasions the exact cause of death is difficult to find, but in general terms it is due to an abnormal reaction by the patient to certain anaesthetic agents. The temperature of the patient steadily rises and may lead to death. The successful treatment of the condition depends on its early recognition, the immediate cessation of any surgery and of the anaesthetic agents, intensive cooling and the institution of the appropriate treatment. The interest in malignant hyperpyrexia is twofold.

First, it is genetically determined; and second, it is a disease caused solely by the administration of medical substances. Because of the genetic association, on recovery from an incident strongly suggestive of the condition, the patient must be investigated to confirm or disprove the diagnosis. If the tests prove positive, then his relatives will also need to be investigated, in case they too have to receive an anaesthetic in the future.

INJURY AND DEATH FROM BURNING

Natural causes

A fairly common cause is *non-ionizing solar radiation*, better known as the sun's rays, which can cause sunburn. It can vary from a mild warm sensation on the skin to a moderately painful experience. It may be suffered by all, to some degree, who unwisely expose large areas of normally covered and 'unhardened' skin to the fierce rays of the sun, either directly or by reflection, for long periods at a time.

There is now an artificial form of sunshine in the form of ultra-violet and infra-red sun lamps, and mild to moderate burns can result from these aids if they are not used in accordance with the maker's instructions.

People with a fair complexion who are in the sun, unprotected, for long periods, may experience severe painful second degree burns with blister formation. The author has seen one such case on a man at a campsite. He was severely sunburnt and had developed an enormous blister which involved the whole of his bald scalp. As a consequence he was in a moderate degree of shock.

A more dramatic cause of burning from a physical agent is that of *lightning*. The most important point to remember is that not all those who have the misfortune to be involved in some way with a stroke of lightning will, necessarily, be killed. There are many examples of people who have been affected by the close proximity of lightning who have recovered completely, or have recovered but with some residual damage to the nervous system.

Because the whole scenario is dramatic, almost every incident of death or injury from lightning becomes immediate national news, but the spectrum of circumstances and patterns of injury are very wide and each case must be considered on its own merits.

It is necessary to have an idea of the general principles involved in a lightning strike. An enormous electrical discharge suddenly passes between an electrically charged layer on the under-surface of a cloud formation and the earth beneath it. Such a discharge generates an enormous amount of heat which rapidly heats up the air surrounding the electrical pathway to an excessively high temperature. The heated air rapidly expands, sending out an omnidirectional shock wave of compressed air. The sudden movement of compressed, superheated air leaves behind a vacuum into which some air must return and then is further released. This then sets up an oscillatory movement of compressed and decompressed air. Such a movement is noisy and accounts for the accompanying thunder.

To any person standing in the range of the oscillating air movement, one or more things may happen. At close proximity to the electrical discharge, the effects are explosive, causing a range of injuries to the body and usually accompanied by destruction of some of the person's clothing. Burns are to be found on the side of the body facing the direction of the blast wave. They are often severe with evidence of scorching or even charring. Further away from the lightning stroke, the burning will be less severe, but will probably show surface 'flash' burns. These may have a linear pattern or an arborescent or 'feathered' pattern. They are similar to first and second degree burns.

Depending on the distance from the stroke, metallic objects on the body become heated to varying degrees. Some may become softened and leave 'metallic' burns on the skin. In other cases, the heating may be less but result in the metal becoming strongly magnetized. This last feature is proof that the injuries received were due to lightning and not from some personal assault or an accident with a fire.

In addition to causing degrees of burning, the blast wave of air has a compression effect, often described by victims as 'having been struck about the head by a heavy object'. The main effect felt is usually on the head, resulting in partial or total loss of consciousness. But the effect may also be felt on the chest or on the abdomen, causing difficulty in breathing or a severe abdominal cramp sensation. The blast effect travels into the body cavities, resulting in internal tissue damage to a variable degree. In extreme cases there may be organ rupture, but more likely it will cause intra-alveoli pulmonary haemorrhage and oedema, or gastro-intestinal bleeding.

As yet the electrical effects on the brain and central nervous system are not fully understood, being similar to the effects of electrocution. What is of importance to all professional workers is that recovery in an apparently dead person is possible, even after an inordinately long period. This means that artificial respiration, of any type, should be continued long after the time when, in other cases, it would seem reasonable to assume that life is extinct.

Dry heat

Burns due to fires, for example, house fires and industrial fires, are very commonplace. Because of their frequency and the complicating factor of inhaling the accompanying smoke, this subject has been fully discussed elsewhere (Chapter 10).

However, there are other sources of dry heat with which contact may be made, especially in the home. The kitchen is particularly important with the oven, the pressing-iron and the central heating boiler being prime examples. Children are particularly liable to receive burns and these may vary from a painful red area to full-thickness skin loss, leading to resultant scar formation.

Moist heat

Burning the body by contact with hot liquids is termed scalding. Scalds in the home are usually caused by boiling water and are most frequently seen in children and in the elderly. The scald only affects the superficial layers of the skin; there is no deeper penetration as with burning. Scalds are recognized by a uniform reddening of the skin and blister formation but with no singed hairs. There may also be red 'trickle' marks due to the flow of the liquid over the body.

However when hot liquids other than boiling water are involved such as super-heated steam, hot fat, jam, industrial fluids, hot oil or even molten metal, then a greater depth of injury will result with full-thickness skin loss and even down to the subcutaneous tissues.

Although scalds are usually superficial, and often localized to a small area of the body, thereby not giving rise to serious concern, on a large scale, scalds can be life-threatening. The signs of shock, infection of the wounds, and tissue fluid loss can all occur in the same manner as with burns, and these complications can cause death.

When large scalds appear on a child, or an elderly, partially mobile, person it is necessary to study the site and distribution of the scalds, bearing in mind at all times that their appearance may not be due to an accident. There may be grounds for regarding the injuries or the death of the person as due to homicide, or attempted homicide. A clue to the true cause may be found if parts of the victim normally held by an attendant, when lowering the person into the water, for example, under the knees, or the upper part of the back, show no scalding, because those parts were held above the water. When boiling water is thrown over a person, the presence and distribution of trickle marks will be of immense importance in determining how the act was carried out, and from which direction.

Radiation

Burns caused by the effects of radiation are important but not frequently encountered. Mention was made above of one form of radiation burn, namely, the sun lamp in association with sunburns.

The worst examples ever seen were undoubtedly burns of enormous severity following the atomic bomb explosions of 1945. Apart from skin lesions, the effects of this form of radiation involved many deeper-seated organs, including the bone marrow.

Other, much less dramatic, cases of radiation burns may follow abnormal exposure to X-rays as well as beta and gamma rays. The results will range from reddening of the skin to full-thickness skin damage extending to the underlying tissues.

More modern forms of radiation are potentially dangerous, if used other than in accordance with the manufacturer's instructions, or if the machines are faulty. These include microwave appliances and laser equipment (Light Amplification by Stimulated Emission of Radiation). The latter may cause localized deep charring of the skin as well as other damage to underlying tissues.

BURNS FROM CHEMICAL AGENTS

Whilst the agents can be subdivided into acids, alkalis and corrosive fluids, each having its own specific chemical properties, they can all cause damage to the skin and even the deeper tissues, resembling the damage caused by heat. As a general rule the chemical agents, in damaging the skin, do not produce any heat, with the exception of sulphuric acid. When this acid comes in contact with the tissue fluids, after destroying the overlying skin, a chemical reaction takes place, generating a considerable amount of heat. Thus the acid with heat results in severe tissue damage.

The other well known mineral acids, and the caustic alkalis, in particular sodium and potassium hydroxide, cause surface tissue destruction and often deep tissue damage without any heat.

In past years the corrosive agents of phenol, lysol and cresol were widely used in various forms of disinfectants and often produced tissue damage both on the surface, and if swallowed. Phenol was particularly dangerous, because when splashed on the skin, it could, if left untouched, produce skin ulceration, which became painless. This was because the phenol attacked the ends of the nerves in the skin and caused local anaesthesia. On occasions phenol was rapidly absorbed into the blood stream and affected the central nervous system, sometimes with fatal results.

The results of accidental contact with chemical agents can be serious, and sometimes produce disfiguring scars. If these occur near joints there is a strong possibility that there will be a marked diminution in articular movement. Such contractures frequently require plastic surgery for correction.

ELECTRICAL INJURIES

WHEN one considers the enormous number of electrical appliances used throughout the country, often by people with scant knowledge or scant regard for the potential danger that exists, it is a matter of surprise that there are not more accidents and fatalities from contact with electricity. Great credit must be given to the manufacturers for their exceedingly high standards of workmanship that allow us all to use electrical appliances with impunity and without harm.

Nevertheless fatalities do occur, even amongst trained electricians. In most cases, judging from conclusions reached by courts of enquiry into each of the deaths, the death is due to careless behaviour, or a poor regard for the customary code of practice.

Example A young electrician, working alone in a home, wished to use his power drill but realized the 13 amp plug on the wire was unsuitable for the 15 amp wall socket. He pulled off the plug and inserted the bare wires into the holes in the wall socket, holding them in place with match-sticks. One of the wires fell out and, it is presumed that whilst trying to re-insert it and hold it in place with the match he accidentally electrocuted himself.

In industry a much higher power supply is in operation for switchgear, heavy power tools etc., requiring a higher degree of skill in maintenance, because there is a higher risk factor involved.

Factors influencing the effect of electricity

(i) *Disease*   Many deaths have been reported in people suffering a variety of chronic debilitating diseases, the contributory factors for the most part remaining largely unknown. However, what is certain is that workers with long-standing heart disease may suffer severe effects, even death, from relatively low tension electrical shocks.

(ii) *Anticipation of a shock*   If one deliberately and consciously sets out to receive a shock, the anticipation of it in some way is a valuable, but not infallible protection. For example, the farmer who deliberately touches the live 'electric fence' which surrounds the field will get an unpleasant shock up his arms. However, if he unwittingly walks into the fence and is, therefore, unprepared for the shock, the result appears to him to have been several times worse.

> *Example*   A man who was accustomed to give himself electrical shocks, by making contact with a 50-volt lamp, performing this act for a wager, made an accidental and unexpected contact with the same lamp – and died! (Taylor, 1965).

(iii) *Voltage*   In the UK and in many places on the continent of Europe the voltage is between 220–240 volts. Other countries, such as Belgium and the USA, have a lower voltage, of 110 volts. The higher voltage produces a larger number of fatalities, probably because it is the commonest voltage in use.

221

Accordingly the even higher voltages, such as are
caused by high tension cables or pylon lines, will increase the risk of death. Accidents occur when
cranes, or metal projections on high vehicles touch
the wires when the vehicles are being moved, or when
people climb pylons for vandalism or to commit
suicide.

There are some notable exceptions. A boy aged 15
years survived after making a suicidal attempt by
touching 8000 volts. In another case a man survived
contact with a wire carrying 4000 volts, but later he
died from a tetanus infection of his injuries.

(iv) *Amperage* This is probably the most important
factor to be considered as regards the electricity itself. A sensation is felt at a level as low as 1mA, being
decidedly unpleasant at a level of 10mA. Between
10mA and 20mA a victim may not be able to release
his hold of the source of electricity, the muscles being
in a condition of intense cramp. This means that he
will receive an electrical current for a long period of
time unless help can be obtained quickly. As the current reaches 50mA–60mA the grip is lost, there is a
loss of muscle control and asphyxia may result from
loss of activity in the respiratory muscles. If the current at this level is maintained for longer than two
seconds, ventricular fibrillation may result. A level of
100mA, received for 0.2 second, will probably be
fatal. The danger obviously increases up to 4A. At
this very high level of 4A, the current is less dangerous than one of 100–150mA. If the heart is fibrillating
and in danger of cessation, a current above 4A may
arrest the fibrillation and return the heart to normal
rhythm. Such is the principle of the treatment with a
defibrillator, used with great success in coronary care

units and resuscitation wards in the hospitals.

(v) *Resistance of the body*   The basic rule in electricity is that the current flowing along a conductor is dependent on the voltage of the electrical source and the resistance of the conductor. Thus we have the well known equation:

$$\text{Current} = \frac{\text{Potential difference in volts}}{\text{Resistance in ohms}}$$

Applying this to the body, the resistance of the skin of the body can vary according to the prevailing conditions.

The thick leathery skin on the heavy workers' palms has a greater resistance than the thinner, softer skin forming the web between his fingers, and even more so when one considers the soft skin of the abdomen.

Similarly the resistance of a dry skin may lie between 2000 and 3000 ohms, but the same skin when wet may only have a resistance of 500 ohms.

The skin has the greatest resistance because at the surface it has the least amount of circulating blood and tissue fluid, both having, by comparison, very little resistance.

(vi) *Earthing*   For electricity to have harmful effects it must flow across or through the body, and to do so the current must be connected to the earth in the same way. To prevent this happening the body must be insulated. Where the insulation is poor or nonexistent the current will flow. Examples of poor or no insulation include standing on damp ground or in wet footwear, and shoes with steel protective fillings increase the danger.

223

(vii) *Electrical path*   There is a greater risk to the person if the heart or the brain lie in the path of current. Examples are a passage from arm to arm, from head to foot or from one arm to the opposite foot.

Cause of death

This is still largely unknown despite animal experimentation, because often death is delayed by a matter of hours. The most important factor is thought to be ventricular fibrillation, especially if the passage of the current involves the chest cavity. But current passing across the chest may cause prolonged muscular contractions of the muscles of respiration, leading to respiratory failure. Sometimes prolonged convulsions occur and this may lead to an asphyxial-like death although, it must be said, the classical signs of asphyxia are usually absent. Some deaths are undoubtedly due to a profound injury to the central nervous system, which is, after all, an electrically based system, so that an excess surge of current would totally disrupt the system.

Signs of death by electrocution

The term usually used to describe the skin lesion is an electrical mark. It may be relatively trivial, or it may be accompanied with a peripheral burn.

There are 3 forms of electrical marks:

(i) *Contact mark*   As the name implies there is a firm

sustained contact with a 'live' object. It may be small, white or yellow with a red margin and possibly with minimal charring.

(ii) *Spark mark*   The mark or marks are due to poor contact with very dry skin. The marks may be multiple, small and scattered due to 'sparking' of the contact on the dry skin. The scattered white marks with poor reddened borders may require microscopic study to provide proof of electrocution.

(iii) *Flash marks*   This is unusual but when it occurs it produces a fine red/yellow arborescent pattern to the skin with accompanying red blotches. It is seen following contact with high voltage.

The exit marks are often difficult to see. If there has been a large area of contact, such as bare feet on a wet floor, then there is nothing abnormal seen. However sometimes exit wounds are found and these take on the form of splits or craters in the skin and underlying tissues – signs of tissue disruption. But in the author's experience, exit wounds are hard to find.

Metallization of the skin may occur at the entry site. This is due to copper (yellow/green) or iron (brown/black) pigments being deposited in the skin.

Example   A student committed suicide following failure in his physics examination. He placed bare copper wires around his wrists and ankles and connected them to a 13 amp plug in a domestic socket. There was marked yellow/green circular marks around the limbs from metallization.

On occasions death from electrocution may be difficult to prove from the examination of the body alone. There may be no abnormal marks to the skin.

An example of this is when electrocution occurs in water, as when an electric appliance falls into a bath of water. The cause of death is then established as much from the circumstances as from the negative autopsy findings.

STARVATION AND NEGLECT

FROM time to time, cases of death from starvation are reported, and usually receive nationwide media coverage. The diagnosis is made from the general severe wasting of the victim or from the unusual circumstances in which the body is discovered, or more usually from a combination of both features.

Deaths from starvation can occur in any of the following circumstances.

Neglect on the part of parents or guardians

Occasionally, as a feature of non-accidental injury in children, there is an associated element of severe neglect. The violence may stop and a neglect to oversee the welfare of the child supersedes. Not only is there starvation but there is usually a supervening infection and inadequate clothing and heating so that death inevitably follows. On occasions there is abnormal mentality in one or other of the parents or the child may be severely retarded, so that there is no real parent–child relationship and a vicious circle results.

Wilful withholding of food

This may be part of the foregoing description of neglect, but deliberate withholding of food is usually a form of punishment or threat and is sometimes seen in relation to the abuse of the elderly. A few years ago the term 'battered grannies' was coined in which the abuse of the very elderly appeared in various forms. Because of the old person's behaviour or habits which were possibly antisocial to the rest of the family, one form of punishment was the deliberate withholding of food. If the state of health of the victim was precarious, continued withholding of food could easily precipitate that state into one of starvation.

Wilful refusal to take food

The condition is one usually associated with females and may be seen amongst the elderly and adolescent girls. The former age group is frequently linked with a paranoid state of fear that the food has been poisoned by other members of the family, or that there is an unreasonable belief that certain basic foods will lead to a fatal disease.

Amongst adolescent girls the desire to remain slim, by restricting the intake of food, may take on a psychological disorder which regards almost all food as abhorrent and dangerous. The state is termed anorexia nervosa, or 'the slimmer's disease' to the popular press. Unless the patient receives prompt, vigorous treatment and psychiatric counselling, the victim can die from starvation.

Entombment

Examples of persons becoming entombed in collapsed mine shafts, old wells and pits or becoming lost in extremely isolated places and succumbing to starvation are reported from time to time. Death is probably the result of a number of factors, including lack of water, lack of air and injury as well as starvation.

Famine

Recent widespread reports from famine-stricken lands in many countries in Africa and to a lesser extent elsewhere, accompanied by photographic evidence, have brought home to the wealthy nations the bald fact that people can still die from famine. However, thankfully it is not something experienced in the UK or Western Europe.

WILFUL NEGLECT OF CHILDREN

WILFUL neglect of children is usually accompanied by some measure of imperfect nutrition, but it usually falls short of starvation. Various Children's and Young Persons' Acts and the Social Work (Scotland) Act 1968 (re-enacting the provisions of the Childrens' Act 1948), covers in Part I the various services available for child care and welfare. They also give advice and assistance to those who are in need of it through the social work department of the local authority.

The main features of wilful neglect are:

1   Failure to provide adequate food;
2   Failure to provide adequate clothing;
3   Failure to provide medical aid;

4   Failure to provide lodging for the child or children in the care of a responsible person.

If a parent or a guardian is unable for whatever reason to provide these basic necessities for the child, then he must apply to the local authority's social work department for them to make the necessary provisions.

Evidence of neglect depends usually on the state of cleanliness and clothing of the child and the general state of nutrition. All children become dirty and untidy, as part of their play and this is obviously within the general knowledge of the visitor, be he doctor, nurse or other professional worker. However, permanently thin, unkempt, imperfectly clad children, bearing in mind the climatic conditions, with a filthy condition of the skin and clothing, a verminous state of the body and hair, with marks of chronic scratching or ulceration, or even a disease of the skin, are all signs of poor parental care. These conditions, when found, may be accepted as sufficient evidence of general neglect, subject to any plausible explanation to the contrary.

Malnutrition is also a sign of neglect and may be obvious. It is definitely established when an accurate description and assessment of the amount of body fat is made together with the height and weight and all these parameters are compared to figures published for average children of similar age.

In the case of a death, the post mortem findings will be directed to the presence of any disease and whether the disease caused the emaciation. It must not be overlooked that diminished nutrition may have been a factor in the causation of certain diseases. The very difficult question for the pathologist is to differentiate cause and effect. In the absence of

229

any disease, there would be grounds for inferring that the death of the child was due to inadequate nourishment.

In assessing wilful neglect by a responsible person, accurate notes regarding the state of housing, in particular the degree of warmth and dryness of the rooms, should be made, along with the amount and variety of food available to the child and the amount and suitability of clothing for the child. In summary, an inventory should be made of all the material factors which have any bearing on the welfare of the apparently neglected child.

Finally, before allegations of wilful neglect can be substantiated, it will be necessary for all persons concerned, including the child himself, to be medically assessed as to their mental condition and consequently their suitability for maintaining a child–adult relationship. If the whole environment is quite unsuitable it will be incumbent on the local authority to remove the child from the home and re-instate him or her in a suitable place of care.

INJURY DUE TO EXPLOSIONS

FREQUENT reports of explosions with details of casualties are becoming part of modern day living. The explosions range in size and effect from the use of sophisticated bombs by terrorist organizations down to domestic gas explosions and even to small blasts caused by schoolchildren experimenting with chemicals.

The nature of the explosive device can vary. Terrorist bombs usually contain commercial gelignite, or a less complex mixture of sodium chlorate and a carbon-containing substance such as sugar. For maximum effect the explosive mixture needs to be tightly packed into a strong metal container such as a beer keg, a gas cylinder or a milk churn. The bomb can then be detonated by one of several methods using a delay mechanism, or even by radio control.

Industrial explosions can also cause widespread and serious damage and often depend on some form of ignition in a gas-filled environment, or an atmosphere of fine dust such as coal, flour or sawdust. If the explosion occurs in an underground tunnel the blast wave will travel very rapidly along the tunnel for a long distance or until it can escape into the atmosphere. Thus injuries can be caused to people working a long way from the origin of the blast.

Example Two men were working on a lining wall in a tunnel which was 212 feet long. At one end of the tunnel there was a 80-foot ventilation shaft which passed straight up to the surface. An explosion occurred approximately 150 feet along the tunnel from the shaft. Three men died in the explosion. The two men who were in the tunnel were three-quarters of the way along from the shaft and the third man was in the shaft. He received severe burns on his back, but managed to climb to the top and he died later. Other people on the surface close to the opening of the shaft were blown off their feet by the blast.

All explosions produce the same results albeit in varying degrees of intensity. There is a blast wave of compressed heated air, flame, smoke and flying fragments. The injuries sustained by the victim will depend entirely on the position of his body to the blast and the distance from it.

231

Blast injuries can be conveniently subdivided into a number of groups but inevitably there will be found a combination of groups or, at least, some overlap of the features.

Total body destruction

This most devastating result is relatively uncommon. It implies that the victim was holding the explosive device, or in extremely close proximity to the explosive source. When the explosion occurred the body caught the full force of the blast, literally blowing the body to pieces. Some of the smaller fragments may be scattered over a very wide area. In fact, some of the pieces necessary for a positive identification may never be found.

Injuries due to the explosion itself

The resulting injuries depend on the force of the explosion, the closeness of the body and the position of the body to the blast wave, and the protection offered by clothing or equipment used. Many victims may suffer the loss of a limb or part of a limb, or the head may be grossly disfigured. These injuries infer close proximity. As the distance increases from the epicentre of the blast, the energy of the blast wave decreases so that the injuries may comprise abrasions, bruises, lacerations or even puncture wounds. Discolouration of the skin by smoke and particulate matter may tattoo or 'pepper' the skin.

INJURIES FROM OTHER SOURCES

Injuries from flying missiles

When the explosion occurs there will be fragments of the container itself which disintegrates together with secondary missiles caused by the blast wave. Thus primary and secondary missiles can produce severe injuries. Secondary missiles may consist of masonry, splintered timber, shattered glass, split corrosive fluid containers or twisted metallic objects. These missiles by reason of their consistency and shape may cause more injury than the primary blast wave. If a body is recovered dead from a collapsed house, the precise cause of death may be difficult to ascertain.

Burns

An explosion generates a very great amount of heat which results in flame and superheated air. The combined effect can result in extensive body burns and burned clothing. The injuries can be similar to those seen on victims of lightning stroke; it is, after all, a similar mechanism.

Equally the explosion can cause a secondary fire, so that if the victim is trapped below collapsed property which is the seat of a fire, serious or fatal burns will result, making it impossible to distinguish primary explosion burns from secondary fire burns.

Effects of the blast wave

The victim may have been positioned so that he/she avoided any direct injury from the flame and flying objects, yet still received severe internal injuries. An explosion produces a wave of very highly compressed air. It may pass out from the source in a ring formation, as seen when a stone is thrown into water or, more probably, the blast wave may be directed along a unique path, sparing objects lying in a different direction, yet still close to the source. In fact, the pathway of the blast wave is largely unpredictable.

A person standing in the pathway of the blast wave will receive the shock on the surface of the body which will then either pass through the solid tissues such as muscle or liver or it may pass through air- or gas-filled cavities such as lung or intestine. In addition the shock wave may pass directly down the trachea and oesophagus to reach the lungs and stomach by a direct route. The internal damage is variable but, in principle, there is an internal shearing effect to the tissues at the interface between air and the tissue. Haemorrhages of varying sizes will occur, sometimes severe enough to fill the alveoli of the lungs or produce a marked gastro-intestinal haemorrhage.

One organ that always suffers some damage following an explosion, even of limited size, is the ear. The blast can cause damage to the ear drum ranging from marked reddening of the surface to actual rupture. There is accompanying intense pain and deafness.

Blast wave injuries may be misdiagnosed, or even pass undetected initially, because there may be nothing to see externally on the victim. All blast wave victims need to be hospitalized with special intensive care, in order that an accurate assessment of the damage can be made.

What caused death?

In all the noise and confusion, dust, debris and carnage, the serious question must be addressed as to why the victim died. Clearly if a dead body is removed from the rubble of a building or mine shaft, it is reasonable to accept that the death was due to the explosion. But to be certain may prove difficult. Death may have occurred from the force of the explosion blast, from penetration of the body by flying objects, either fragments of the bomb casing or from secondary missiles. It may have been caused by crush asphyxia from being buried under fallen timber or masonry. It might also have resulted from a natural cause, such as a heart attack brought on by the shock of the event. The need for a careful post mortem examination is essential if one is to learn anything from the tragic circumstances.

REFERENCE

Taylor, A.S. (1965) *Principles and Practice of Forensic Medicine*, Churchill, London.

10   FIRE CASUALTIES

OVER the past 40 years throughout the UK the annual number of fires occurring in occupied buildings has remained fairly constant, being about 120,000 per year. In contrast, during the same period, there has been a general increase in the total number of casualties, both fatal and non-fatal. Significantly, the percentage of persons overcome by smoke and fire gases has steadily increased by as much as five times, whilst the percentage suffering from burn injuries has decreased.

The apparent increase in deaths due to smoke inhalation may be as a result of improved laboratory techniques, allowing for a more readily available analysis and measurement of the fire gases, but equally, it may be argued that there is now an increased awareness by pathologists that the death of a fire victim is more likely to be attributed to smoke and fire gases rather than to the effects of body burns.

There is a general concern by medical and scientific workers that the rise in the number of fire deaths due to smoke and gas intoxication reflects closely the increased use of synthetic polymers, the 'plastics', in the modern home; materials for construction, furniture, household goods and internal decoration. Laboratory studies on many of the commonly used plastics have shown that excessive quantities of smoke and highly toxic decomposition products are formed during the burning and heat destruction of the materials. It is noteworthy that the speed with which the fire develops is now much more rapid than in former 'non-plastic' times, and the ease with which the plastics ignite coupled with their rapid rate of burning is probably the cause of more rapidly produced injury, or even death, to the fire victim.

The majority of the fire deaths occur in dwelling houses, usually the living room or the bedroom where the fire is relatively small in size. The result is usually a single fatality and is frequently associated with some domestic activity close to the fire, or to some personal activity, such as smoking a cigarette in bed.

THE HAZARDS OF A FIRE

BEFORE considering the pathological and toxicological aspects of a fire fatality, it is necessary to consider briefly the main life-threatening factors of a domestic fire.

Oxygen depletion

The rapid consumption of oxygen mostly produces carbon dioxide, which in high concentration alone is life-threatening, but also carbon monoxide and other gases in variable amounts. The level of oxygen available to the victim trapped in a fire atmosphere depends on the quantity of the combustible materials present, the rate of burning, the volume of the confined space and the adequacy of any ventilation present. An oxygen concentration of less than 10 per cent is believed to be insufficient to sustain life.

Flame and heat burns

Burns, heat stroke, shock, dehydration and tissue oedema can all be caused by direct contact with, or radiation heat from, the flame. Breathing in a very hot environment can be extremely difficult and painful, and can damage the lining of the respiratory tract.

Temperatures attained in fires are frequently very high; for example temperatures of 600°–800°C can be reached in a dwelling house fire in 5 to 15 minutes. In some exceptional fires temperatures of 1000°C can be reached in only two minutes. Such rapidly produced high temperatures play a part in preventing the occupants of a burning house from reaching fire exit doors.

Smoke

Smoke is defined as the mixture of airborne substances produced when a material is decomposed by heat or burning. Smoke may contain gases, liquids, solid particles or a combination of these. Apart from reducing visibility, smoke brings about an intense irritation to the eyes and mucous membrane of the respiratory tract. This is because irritant and toxic substances such as hydrochloric acid are absorbed on to the smoke particles.

Smoke also contributes to confusion, a state of disorientation and panic. As the smoke becomes denser, it will hinder or even prevent the escape of the occupants as well as the entry of the rescuers. In some places smoke can reach unacceptable levels, in terms of toxicity and optical density, long before the temperature does.

Destruction of the building

As the fire increases in size the fabric of the building, as opposed to the contents, will be damaged or destroyed, rendering various parts of it unsafe. Falling ceilings and collapsing floors to be followed by larger items such as beams, joists and even masonry can contribute to the worsening state of the victim, either by injuring him directly or trapping him under the weight of the objects, or even by blocking his escape route.

THE MEDICO-LEGAL ASPECTS OF A FIRE DEATH

THE problem to be faced by the investigating police and fire officers is this: did the person die before the fire started? or did the person die because of the fire?

If the person died *before* the fire started, did he die from some natural cause, such as a heart attack or an internal haemorrhage and in dying did he fall against a source of heat, causing his clothes and body to burn and as a consequence the fire spread to involve the surrounding area?

An alternative suggestion might be that he died from some unnatural cause, such as homicide, and the fire was then started deliberately to conceal the crime. Over the past ten years, 14 cases of homicide in which fire played a part have been recorded in the Glasgow area. In eight of the cases a fire was started in an attempt to burn the body and cover the injured area. In all cases, the negative pathological and toxicological findings (see below) clearly indicated that death occurred before, or very soon after the start of the fire.

In one case an electrician died from electrocution while stripping wire out of a derelict house, which was believed to have been disconnected from the main supply. While he was still in contact with the wire, a fire was started by a short circuit affecting the nearby dry wood and later the whole room. Pathological examination with toxicological analysis determined that he had died before the fire had started.

If the person died *after* the fire had started then a subsequent post mortem examination will reveal a number of important findings confirming the cause of death. These findings can be divided into pathological findings and toxicological findings.

Pathological findings

(i) *External appearances*   A body recovered from a fire may show very little external damage, amounting to no more than a fine deposition of soot particles on the exposed areas. Many cases, however, show burns to the skin ranging from mere reddening and some early blister formation to extensive damage with charring. Frequently, however, when there has been a delay in recovering the body, the prolonged exposure to the heat causes the body to adopt a characteristic 'pugilistic' attitude, once interpreted as a 'fleeing from the fire' posture. This is a typical post mortem appearance. It is caused by the heat producing a greater contraction of the flexor muscles than the extensor muscles. The effect is seen in the arms, wrists and hands, resembling a boxer's stance, and in the muscles of the thighs, lower legs and feet which simulate a 'fight or flight' position (see Figure 10.1).

An additional finding over the large muscle groups is the presence of linear splits in the skin which may resemble incised wounds. They are caused by the expansion of the fat and muscle and the tissue fluid under a tense skin.

It is well to remember that no matter how badly charred and disfigured a body may appear, the internal organs are usually extremely well preserved and therefore fully amenable to a post mortem examination.

(ii) *Burn injuries* The severity of a burn injury in the living as well as the dead may be determined either in terms of the area of body surface affected, or in terms of the depth of a wound. In the former case the assessment can be made with reference to the 'rule of nines', whereby the body is arbitrarily divided into multiples of nine up to 100 per cent (see Figure 10.2). On the other hand burns may be classified as deep or superficial depending on whether or not the full thickness of the skin has been destroyed and if it has, then to what extent the deeper structures are affected.

In a study of fire deaths in Glasgow, 82 per cent of the fire victims had burn injuries and in 62 per cent

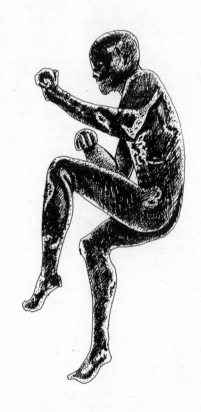

FIGURE 10.1   CHARACTERISTIC
'PUGILISTIC' ATTITUDE CAUSED BY
PROLONGED EXPOSURE TO HEAT

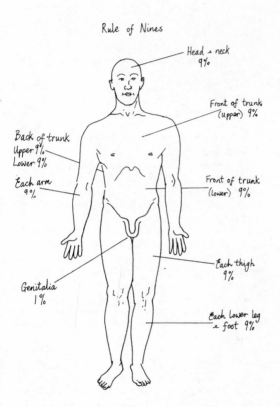

Rule of Nines

Head & neck
9%

Front of trunk
(upper) 9%

Back of trunk
Upper 9%
Lower 9%

Each arm
9%

Front of trunk
(lower) 9%

Genitalia
1%

Each thigh
9%

Each lower leg
& foot 9%

**FIGURE 10.2   DIVISION OF BODY
ACCORDING TO THE 'RULE OF NINES'**

the burns were so extensive as to involve most of the body surface. When skin is damaged to that extent any evidence of the important 'vital reaction' sign, a characteristic reddening at the edge of an injury, indicating that the victim was alive when the burn was sustained, is largely destroyed.

Whether or not a burned victim survives, allowing for other factors found in a fire, will depend largely on the extent of the burned area, rather than on its site and depth. Whilst there are exceptions, it is generally understood that if more than 40 per cent of the body is involved the chances of survival are poor, and if over 60 per cent the chances are nil. Survival at these high percentages depends so much on the promptness and standard of treatment. With modern burns units, surgical teams have achieved remarkable successes.

Following a severe burn the normal sequence of events is first collapse due to neuro-psychological shock, followed by physiological shock, a peripheral vascular collapse due to fluid loss and blood shift. Then may follow a stage of toxaemia. Later complications, in the absence of healing, are infections within the burned areas and bronchopneumonia. More remote complications affect the kidneys, liver and heart.

(iii) *Respiratory tract injuries* The mucous membrane and other deeper structures of the respiratory system are particularly vulnerable to damage from a combination of heat, smoke and fire gases. The Glasgow study showed that in 84 per cent of the deaths there was marked oedema and early inflammation of mucosa and submucosa with frequent shedding of the mucosal lining.

An important finding, and one that is easy to see, is the presence of soot particles on the mucosal surface of the larynx and trachea. Sometimes it is seen as soot mixed with free mucus; at other times the soot appears as large shiny sheets firmly adherent to the trachea. In 92 per cent of the cases studied soot was seen with the naked eye. The respiratory tract injuries have been shown to be produced by both direct exposure to heat and by irritant gases. The heated air causes obstructive oedema to the epiglottis and the vocal cords, but in addition the thermal shock may induce a reflex closure of the larynx, thereby severely restricting breathing. If the victim had inhaled flames as well as smoke there will be scorching and tissue destruction of the pharynx, epiglottis and larynx.

Heat effects are still possible on the deeper parts of the airway if the humidity of the air, and therefore, the heat capacity, is exceptionally high. Small smoke particles may be carried through the smallest bronchi into the bronchioles, and along with them irritant gases. Some cellular shedding, desquamation, may be seen at these deep levels.

The inhaled soot particles may trap irritant materials from the fire on to the surfaces of the bronchioles and when the soot is stopped by the mucous membrane, the irritants, such as hydrogen chloride, nitrogen oxides and aldehydes, may bring about a reflex closure of the bronchioles, similar in effect to a severe attack of asthma. It is uncommon to find soot particles beyond the bronchioles.

(iv) *Injuries to the head*   A frequent finding is that of heat fractures to the skull. These may consist of an irregular linear fracture, a sprung suture or less commonly a stellate fracture and they are usually found involving the parietal bone, often accompanied by herniation of the brain.

In addition, there may be a large extradural heat haematoma which may simulate an ante mortem injury but it is unaccompanied by any other signs suggesting blunt force injury. The haematoma is found where the head has been exposed to intense heat sufficient to cause charring of the skull. In the absence of a skull fracture the distribution of the clot follows closely the outline of the charring of the outer table. The blood clot is not uniformly solid but has a fine honeycombed appearance, the tiny spaces representing former steam bubbles.

Although these artefacts are well recognized, there is still a need to exercise caution before lightly accepting them as mere post mortem incidents.

Toxicologial findings

There are two aspects of the toxicology of fire deaths that must be considered. First, the toxic effects of the smoke and the various fire gases produced by combustion, and second, the contributory effects of alcohol and other drugs taken by the victim before the fire.

(i) *Smoke and fire gases* During the early stages of a fire, there is usually sufficient oxygen in the vicinity to permit complete or almost complete combustion. This results in the formation of carbon dioxide. As the fire develops carbon monoxide, nitrous oxides and hydrogen chloride are formed, and then with further development, oxygen-starved combustion occurs, leading to the formation and release of complex compounds. These include hydrocarbons, hydrogen cyanide, aldehydes and ketones, each contributing to the toxic hazard of the fire.

(ii) *Carbon monoxide*   It has been recognized for a long time that the most important toxic product of a fire is carbon monoxide. It is a colourless and odourless gas which binds itself to haemoglobin in the red corpuscles 300 times more readily than oxygen. This gives rise to a characteristic cherry-pink colour to the blood and soft tissues of the body. The remarkable affinity of carbon monoxide for haemoglobin results in a rapid reduction in the oxygen-carrying capability of the blood with noticeable neurological changes in a very short time. Concentrations of carbon monoxide in blood are usually expressed in terms of the percentage of haemoglobin saturated with the gas, thus %HbCO. The toxic effects as listed in Table 10.1 are very well known. One of the complications of carbon monoxide poisoning is that the rapid onset of muscular incoordination and weakness may seriously impair the speed and direction of the victim's escape.

The level at which carbon monoxide poisoning may be assumed to be fatal is 60%HbCO and over. This will apply to any situation where carbon monoxide is produced, for example, the exhaust fumes of a motor car or a poorly functioning paraffin heater. In a fire, however, there are additional factors such as an elevated carbon dioxide and lowered oxygen levels in the enclosed air which increases the toxic effects of carbon monoxide. Consequently the fatal level of carbon monoxide in a fire fatality is frequently 50%HbCO. Analyses of blood from fire fatalities, in the UK indicate that more than three-quarters of the

TABLE 10.1

TOXIC EFFECT DUE TO CARBON MONOXIDE POISONING

%HbCO	Symptoms
0–10	No noticeable effects
10–20	Shortness of breath and giddiness may be observed during exercise
20–30	Shortness of breath, giddiness, headache even in the absence of exercise
30–50	Muscular control becomes difficult, resulting in incoordination and staggering. Loss of consciousness may be induced by exercise
50–80	Coma, followed by death due to respiratory arrest

deaths are due solely to carbon monoxide poisoning; the remainder involved additional factors.

(iii) *Hydrogen cyanide* This is a thermal degradation product of many nitrogen-containing polymeric materials in both natural materials such as wool, silk and horsehair and in synthetic materials such as polyurethane and polyacrylonitrile.

The cyanide reacts very rapidly with an enzyme found in the mitochondria of cells to form a cytochrome oxidase cyanide complex. The complex inhibits cellular respiration which in turn leads to hypoxia. In quite low concentration cyanide stimulates the respiratory centre in the brain, encouraging deep breathing whilst at the same time cyanide depresses the general electrical activity of the brain. There still remains much uncertainty in the interpretation of cyanide levels obtained from the blood samples in determining the fatal level for cyanide poisoning in association with other gases.

Cigarette smoke contains cyanide gas. The range of cyanide concentrations found in the blood of smokers ranges from 0–20μmol/litre (significantly higher than in non-smokers). From the literature, significant toxic effects, although non-fatal, are experienced with a blood cyanide level of around 50μmol/litre, with a serious risk to life when the level is around 100μmol/litre. In the Glasgow study of fire fatalities, for which cyanide measurements were available, 24 per cent had blood levels likely to produce significant toxic effects (over 50μmol/litre) a quarter of whom had potentially fatal levels (over 100μmol/litre).

(iv) *Other fire gases*   From blood samples of fire fatalities analysed for the presence of organic compounds, a number of substances have been identified and quantified. These include hydrocarbons, carbonyls, nitriles, and heterocyclic compounds. Many of these compounds are highly toxic, e.g. acrolein, and may be significant in affecting the victim during the early stages of exposure to the fire. Their precise role in causing fire deaths has not yet been clearly demonstrated, mainly because of insufficient data relating to blood levels and their toxic effects.

(v) *The abuse of alcohol*   By far the most important contributory non-incendiary factor in fire deaths, as shown by the Glasgow study, is the abuse of alcohol.

In 64 per cent of adults aged 18 years and over there was laboratory evidence suggesting gross intoxication at the outbreak of the fire, with an average post mortem blood level of 229mg alcohol per 100ml blood. More men than women had been drinking alcohol before the fire and this concurs with the Scottish drinking habits which show that 74 per cent of men as against 46 per cent women are regular drinkers.

Drugs such as sedatives, tranquillizers and sleeping tablets, either alone or in conjunction with alcohol, were not found to play a significant factor in the fire deaths. Only a small number of blood samples tested showed the presence of drugs and these were all at therapeutic levels.

Other medico-legal aspects

(i) *Suicide*   Over the past ten years there have been 12 cases of suicide involving fire reported from the Glasgow area. Most of the cases involved pouring paraffin over the head and front of the body and then igniting it. The following case is unusual.

> *Example*   An elderly female in a hospital ward who had just learnt of her diagnosis quietly went to the toilet which opened from a corridor. She was wearing a nightdress only. While in the toilet she placed a pile of toilet paper at her feet and lit it with a match. She stood over the burning paper and allowed the nightdress to catch fire. When well alight she came out of the toilet to collapse in front of a nurse. There had been no noise or appeals for help; she died later from extensive body burns.

An interesting feature of suicide by fire (self-immolation) is the repetitive nature of the action. If the first case has been well publicized then a small series of others may soon follow.

(ii) *Access to exits*   Among other factors which need to be investigated are the ease of access to the door and whether it opens freely, the siting of fire exits and directional signs, the position of the window and whether it opens and the density and opacity of the smoke which increase the difficulty of discovering the exit route.

From the medical standpoint there is a need to know whether the victim had impaired sight or hearing and whether artificial aids were used; the presence of some orthopaedic disability making movements slow and painful, the overwhelming elements of shock surprise and panic; and the age of the victim, the very young and very old being disproportionately more vulnerable than other age groups.

The nature and material of clothing or bedding which may have been set alight following a light contact with a source of heat is of importance especially in view of recent efforts to make children's clothing of a non-flammable material.

From what has been said it follows that there is still a great need for more advice and education to those at greatest risk, namely the aged, infirm and regular users of tobacco and alcohol to the inherent risks which could lead to an outbreak of fire. They must especially be warned of the ease with which many modern materials catch fire and the rate of the spread of the flames which thereby reduce substantially the time in which a person may escape and avoid inhaling dangerous fire products.

REFERENCES

Anderson, R.A., Watson, A.A. & Harland, W.A. (1981), *Med.Sci.Law*, **21**,3, p. 175.
Anderson, R.A., Watson, A.A. & Harland, W.A. (1981), *Med.Sci.Law*, **21**,4, p. 288.

11   FIREARMS AND FIREARM INJURIES

From time to time a police officer, a nurse, or some other professional person may be asked to attend the scene of a shooting accident, and perhaps be asked to express an opinion as to the nature of the injury. If that opinion is to be worth anything, it is essential that the person have an elementary knowledge of the rudiments of ballistics and the types of firearms available, remembering at all times that detailed opinions upon particular firearms and their ammunition, together with the resultant injuries, must be left to a firearms expert.

This chapter seeks to offer a reasonable guide to the interpretation of firearm injuries as well as helping the observer to recognize the common types of weapons available.

A GENERAL CLASSIFICATION OF FIREARMS

The firearms which are more or less readily available to the general public can be divided into two main groups, depending on whether the interior of the barrel of the weapon is smooth or grooved. The inside of the barrel is referred to as the bore, and the grooved or lined appearance of the bore is known as the rifling. Thus we can classify firearms as follows:

1   Smooth-barrelled weapons = 'smooth bore' – airgun, shotgun
2   Rifled or grooved barrels = 'rifled bore' – revolver, automatic pistol, service rifle, sporting rifle.

The indiscriminate use of the word 'gun' by itself is to be deplored, for if the professional person repeatedly refers to 'a gun', it tends to infer a singular lack of understanding of the subject. The word 'gun' is really only used in the composite word 'shotgun'. Although it is not incorrect to use the word 'airgun', it is preferable to be more explicit and describe the weapon as an air pistol or an air rifle.

Air weapons

These smooth-bored weapons, seen as air pistols or air rifles, fire either single small lead pellets, or conical, flighted or lightly feathered darts, by means of compressed atmospheric air. The lead pellets, which are sometimes referred to as slugs, measure about one-fifth of an inch in length. The flighted darts are considerably larger.

For years, these weapons were regarded as little more than toys for schoolboys, or at least as innocent sporting weapons, despite the fact that eye surgeons have long known that a pellet can destroy an eye. Moreover, there are cases on record, albeit rare, of pellets from air weapons having caused death from severe brain damage, so that the idea that these weapons are not dangerous can no longr be substantiated.

Example   An adult who was child-minding was firing an airgun at a target placed on the floor on the opposite side of a kitchen. A child of three years walked across the line of fire and a pellet penetrated his skull in the parieto-temporal region. He developed an epileptic seizure and underwent emergency surgery. An extradural haematoma was removed together with a part of the frontal pole of the cerebral hemisphere which contained the pellet. There was no improvement after surgery and he died shortly afterwards as a consequence of raised intracranial pressure.

Under the Firearms Act, 1968, section 22, ss (4) and (5), it is an offence for a person under the age of 14 to be in possession of an air weapon, or even to have ammunition for it. Persons over 14 may be lent or given an airgun, but it is illegal to sell such a weapon to anyone under the age of 17. The carrying of an airgun in a public place by a person under 17 is prohibited, unless the weapon is securely covered. There are now available some especially dangerous air weapons, defined as pump-action air rifles with a high kinetic energy, and these are classified as 'Section 1' firearms, for which a firearms certificate is required.

Shotguns

Although these weapons may have only one barrel, most sportsmen and farmers prefer to have the double-barrelled version, the two barrels usually lying side by side. On the continent, one will frequently find one barrel lying above the other. However, the overall length of all shotguns lies between 40 and 48 inches.

While outwardly the two barrels appear identical, the interiors are different. That of the right, or upper barrel, is usually a true cylinder; but that of the left, or lower barrel, is narrowed, or 'choked' for a part of its length adjoining the muzzle. The purpose of choking is to pack the shot charge into a more compact harder-hitting mass, effective at a longer range than the shot charge from an ordinary, unchoked, barrel.

Three grades of choke are used, and these are termed 'improved cylinder', narrowing by 3 to 5 thousands of an inch; 'half choke', narrowing by 15 to 20 thousands of an inch, and full choke, narrowing by 35 to 40 thousands of an inch. The normal muzzle velocity for a shotgun is of the order of 1000 feet per second, and the lethal range for game birds and animals, depending on the degree of choke, is normally between 30 and 40 yards.

The calibre of large shotguns is expressed according to their bore, or barrel diameter. For example a sportsman will describe his weapon as a '12-bore' or a '16-bore' shotgun. The description is archaic and quaint and has little practical value, but nevertheless the terms are still in general use.

The size of the bore is determined by the number of lead spheres, each identical to the other, and each of which will precisely fit the barrel, that can be made from 1lb of lead. For example, a 12-bore shotgun will have a larger diameter than as 16-bore because only 12 balls can be made from the 1lb of lead large enough to fit the barrel, whereas with the smaller

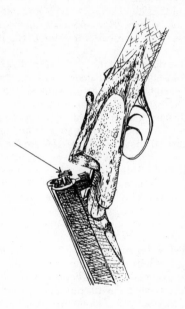

FIGURE 11.1   A HIGH-GRADE DOUBLE-
BARRELLED SPORTING GUN OPEN READY
FOR LOADING

diameter, a 16-bore weapon, 16 smaller balls can be made to fit its barrel from the same amount of lead.

In modern terms, each of the 12 lead balls has a diameter of 0.729in. Therefore a 12-bore gun has a diameter of 0.729in. But nobody remembers the actual barrel size – it is easier to think of the 12 lead balls.

When the diameter of the barrel is less than half an inch the old classification does not apply and the calibre is given by that diameter. Thus another common, smaller, sporting gun is known as the '410'. It has a single barrel, the bore being 0.410in or 11mm.

It is well to remember that some criminals may carry a sawn-off shotgun. The barrels are inexpertly shortened by sawing them across, usually about one-third of the way from the breech. This allows the weapon to be concealed inside a coat. Sawing off a barrel indiscriminately will render the weapon inacurate, but it is still very dangerous.

With regard to the ammunition that is used for the shotgun, whatever its size, the various components detailed below remain proportionally the same. It consists of a cylinder of waterproofed cardboard, or polythene, mounted in a brass head, into which is set, at the base, a small detonator cap. The cap is made of copper and holds a small amount of an explosive substance, usually fulminate of mercury. When the cap is struck by the firing pin, this substance immediately ignites. Within the lower quarter or so of the cylinder is situated the main explosive powder, which in turn is ignited by the detonator. The main powder varies with different makes of ammunition, but nitrocellulose or nitroglycerine is usually incorporated.

The main explosive powder is covered by a wad of rubber, plastic or felt. This prevents the main wad lubricant coming into contact with the powder, as well as protecting the main wad from the burning powder.

Above the felt wad lies the main propellant wad. It cushions the shot from the initial impact of the explosion as well as conserving the power of the exploding powder behind it until the pressure builds up to a maximum.

Finally, above the main wad, and perhaps separated from it by a further thin wad, lies the collection of lead shot which can be obtained in various sizes or diameters depending on the size of game for the hunter. The free edge of the cartridge case is then closed over the shot to keep the pellets in place, and a thin waterproof or waxed disc is inserted.

In passing, it is of some interest, in this highly techical age, to realize that lead shot is still made in the traditional way, in a 'shot-tower'. Molton lead alloy is poured through a sieve and is allowed to drop into a tank of water 185 feet below. Perfect spherical shot is obtained in various sizes and these are graded to very close limits.

In considering the injuries produced it is worth remembering that the collective term for all injuries caused by firearms is '*gun-shot wounds*', but when the wounds are caused specifically by a popular sporting weapon, such as the 12-bore shotgun, then we must use the term '*a shotgun wound*'.

There are two further points to remember. First, so long as the wads are in contact with the lead shots, then the shots will remain in a compacted mass, but as soon as the effect of the compression drops away, the pellets move away from the wads and begin to fan out. Second, the propellant powder continues burning, producing gases, soot and flame down the entire

length of the barrel. Some powder will remain unburned, so that both soot and unburned powder
travel together for a short distance from the end of
the barrel. These facts can help us to estimate the
distance between the muzzle of the barrel and the
victim.

A muzzle in contact with the skin will produce a
'contact wound'. The diameter of the entry wound
will be the same as the diameter of the barrel.
Around the perimeter of the wound there will be
bruising and some abrasions caused by the recoil of
the weapon. If a double-barrelled gun has been used
there will probably be a circular bruised abrasion
close by, caused by the second barrel. The rim of the
wound shows a backened border, because unburned
powder and soot have been forced into the surrounding skin. The escaping hot gases will also burn the
skin close to the rim of the wound. Any carbon monoxide contained in the hot gases may form local carboxyhaemoglobin, giving to the tissues in the wall of
the wound a characteristically bright pink colour.

The explosive gases entering the wound with the
shot may partly blow back, causing a very ragged
entry wound. If bone is close by, then the whole bony
mass may be shattered. It is the entry of the still-
expanding hot gases that produces such severe destruction to the internal organs.

As the distance from the muzzle to the skin wound
increases, these characteristics diminish; indeed, at
about eight feet tattooing by powder grains is usually
absent and the wads and perhaps the gases fail to
enter the wound. The wound caused by the shot is
irregular in outline. As the distance increases still
more the shot fans out and the central hole becomes
smaller until at about 24 feet there is only a uniform

spread of pellet holes on the skin.

We must not overlook the fact that the diameter of the spread of shot depends on which barrel was fired, the normal one or the choked one. Over a short distance, up to 30 feet, the difference is probably insignificant but beyond this distance it does matter. However, beyond 60 feet it is unlikely that the wound will be fatal.

As a working rule-of-thumb, the mean diameter of the pattern of the shot, when measured in inches, is equal to the distance from the muzzle measured in yards.

We have seen that wounds received from any close range result in extensive internal damage, and an interesting variant of this is seen when the muzzle is placed against the head. The combined effects of expanding gases and lead shot is like an explosion inside the skull, and the top of the head may be totally disintegrated.

The usual sites for suicide wounds are limited in number, because the length of the barrel is almost the same as the length of the arm. That means that there is always some difficulty in reaching the trigger. Suicide wounds are therefore seen in the roof of the mouth, the centre of the forehead, the temples, or in the centre of the chest. They are selected so as to eliminate the possibility of failure.

Rifled firearms

These comprise amongst others the revolver, the automatic pistol, the machine gun and the service and sporting rifles. They all discharge a single projectile – a bullet. The weapons may fire the bullets singly or in rapid fire depending on the mechanism. The calibre or diameter of a bullet may vary in size but generally the bullets are between 0.3 and 0.4in. It is the diameter size that is used when describing an old service rifle, for example. One spoke of a 303 rifle because it fired a bullet 0.303in in diameter. Other calibres are given in inch decimals or in millimetres – '.450', '.380', 11.25mm, 9mm etc., and these figures represent the diameter of the barrel bore before the cutting of the grooves (rifling).

The purpose of the rifling system is to spin the bullet around its longitudinal axis, thus giving it stability in flight and resisting any tendency for the bullet to change its altitude during its flight. Between the grooves cut in the barrel the sections of metal which stand out are termed the *lands* of the barrel. The lands dig into the lead bullet or into the metal jacket of a composite bullet so that when the bullet passes along the bore by the gases, the twist of the lands between the grooves causes the bullet to rotate. As the bullet leaves the muzzle it is travelling at its maximum speed and spinning at its highest rate.

We must at this point remember to use the correct terminology. A bullet is the missile, usually made of lead. It may be jacketed by copper or not. The bullet is held in a cartridge case together with the powder charge and the primer. All the assembled parts form a cartridge. The word cartridge is not the prerogative of the sporting shotgun but is applied to ammunition for all firearms, even though it may sound slightly strange.

The *revolver* is a relatively heavy weapon even when unloaded. It weighs between 1¾ and 2¾lb, and has a barrel length of between 5 and 6½in. Below the barrel there is a cylinder or drum which is fitted with six separate chambers, into each of which a cartridge is inserted (see Figure 11.2). The cylinder revolves around a centre pin; this movement of course gives rise to the name of the weapon. Each time the trigger is released, the cylinder revolves a sufficient distance to bring another cartridge into the breech. After the cartridge has been fired the empty case is not ejected but remains in the cylinder until it is emptied by hand.

The *self-loading or automatic pistol* carries its ammunition in a metal container, the magazine, which is fitted below the breech (see Figure 11.3). When in place it acts as part of the handpiece to the weapon. After a cartridge has been fired, the empty cartridge case is automatically ejected from the side of the breech. The cartridge case may be sent several feet away from where the firer is standing. This is a point of practical importance, because the jettisoning of spent cases after a burst of firing may mean that one or more may be left at the scene, either because the assailant has not had time to retrieve them, or because he was unable to find them.

The cartridge case for the revolver has a base projecting out as a flange which allows the case to remain in the cylinder. On the other hand the cartridge case for the pistol has a groove running round the base into which the ejector pin fits to eject the case from the breech (see Figure 11.4). The ejector pin will mark the case in such a way that an inspection and study of the case mark may help link a particular weapon with the ammunition fired.

The bullet wounds which result from a weapon fired at contact or close range have a similar appearance, albeit very much smaller, to those of a shotgun injury, with bruising, blast effects, the deposition of soot and tattooing.

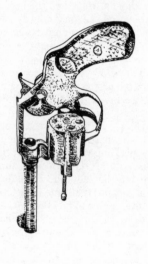

FIGURE 11.2   A REVOLVER OPEN READY FOR LOADING

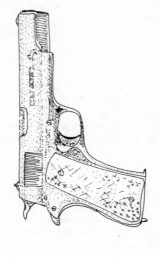

FIGURE 11.3   AN AUTOMATIC PISTOL

The appearance of the wound depends on whether the bullet is in the early part or the last part of the flight, when there is a considerable degree of 'tail-wag'. This wobble causes a relatively large and ragged entry wound. In the intervening part of its flight, the bullet is stable and when it enters a body it will make a clean wound, with a slightly inverted margin, often with a greasy or oily rim, unless the bullet has passed first through clothing which will remove most of the grease.

The exit wound is likely to be irregular and if the flight of the bullet has been disturbed by contact with bone or firm tissue the exit hole may be greatly enlarged with eversion of the skin edge. The bullet may shatter a bone so that there may be exit wounds made by pieces of bone as well as the bullet. The bullet itself might fragment so that more than one small exit wound may be seen.

When a bullet is travelling at a very high speed, as with the modern high velocity rifle, the bullet kills by reason of the release of a very large amount of kinetic energy. As the bullet slows during its passage through the body, shock waves radiate from the bullet's pathway causing large lacerations in organs such as heart, liver and brain with a consequent massive haemorrhage.

Examination of a recovered bullet, even if the bullet is damaged, can help identify the weapon concerned. A test firing is made by the suspect weapon and the test bullet and the recovered bullet are examined side by side by means of a comparative microscope in order to study the markings produced by the rifling of the barrel (see Figure 11.5).

Thus the ejection mark on the side of a cartridge case, the position of the indentation caused by the

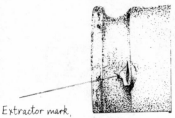

Extractor mark,
Colt Automatic Pistol Caliber .32

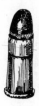

·380 Revolver Cartridge,
straight rimmed case

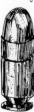

·45 Self loading Pistol
Cartridge, straight rimless
case.

← base

FIGURE 11.4   TYPES OF PISTOL and REVOLVER CARTRIDGES

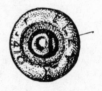

410 shotgun cartridge cases - fired by same gun

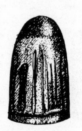

Rifling engraving

FIGURE 11.5   EXAMINATION OF RECOVERED CARTRIDGE CASES AND BULLET

firing pin on the base of the cartridge and the 'land' markings on the bullet are very useful points of evidence in linking a particular weapon with a certain crime, but it must be stressed that this study must be left to the ballistics expert.

There just remains to be mentioned a few other weapons, rarely called into question. They include stud guns and rivet guns in industry, humane killers in abattoirs, starting guns at race meetings, firearms in approved rifle clubs and fairground shooting galleries, and weapons that fire rubber or plastic bullets, or discharge a harmful liquid or gas.

CONSIDERATION OF THE INJURY

THE role of the forensic personnel is to provide assistance in the distinction to be made between suicide, accident or homicide. An examination of the locus will help with regard to suicide. Is the weapon within reach of the deceased, and from the site of the wound could that weapon produce it in the hands of the person himself? On occasions elaborate devices have been set up to fire the weapon because the suicide victim cannot reach the trigger. Such a device will prove most valuable to the investigation.

Accidental and homicidal wounds are often difficult to distinguish. A single wound in the back of the neck or behind the ear is almost certainly homicidal, especially if it is in contact, but other sites may make one less sure. The presence of more than one injury will be very strong evidence against both accident and suicide. In practice the suspicion of homicide rests on the exclusion of suicide by the pathologist, after which the matter will depend on the circumstantial evidence provided by the police. Full background reports on the deceased's mental state, socio-economic situation and knowledge of firearms must be sought to augment the medical and scientific findings before any firm decision can be reached.

12   DEATH IN CHILDHOOD

It is well known that the majority of deaths, both from natural disease and external trauma, apply to children as well as to the adult population. On the other hand, there are sufficient differences in the investigation of infant deaths to warrant a special chapter dealing with problems peculiar to this age group.

THE NEW-BORN INFANT

On examination of a dead infant which appears to have been recently born, a number of questions present themselves.

1   Is it a full-term baby, or is it premature?
2   Is it a stillbirth, or has it breathed?
3   If it breathed, when did it die?
4   Did it die from natural causes?
5   Did it die from inattention?
6   Did it die from some act of violence?

Full-term or premature

It is important to know whether the dead infant was delivered at the end of a normal period of gestation, or whether it is premature – an infant born between the 28th week of gestation and full term – or perhaps it is a foetus of a still earlier period. The answer is obtained first by external factors and then by examination of the internal organs, especially the centres of ossification. The crown–heel length, the crown–rump length and the circumference of the head are measured and the body is weighed. The results are then read off against standard tables prepared for foetuses and infants at certain ages. In addition the state of the fingernails, the descent of the testes and the presence of fine lanugo body hair are noted and checked against the tables.

Internally, apart from the state of development of the organs and systems, the presence of the ossification centres in the lower end of the femur, the cuboid bone of the foot, and the upper end of the tibia will indicate that the child is full-term. Of all the observations made, it is generally accepted that the presence of the ossification centres has the greatest value.

Still-birth or separate existence

Proof that the child has had a separate existence may be obtained by means of an autopsy, because positive external signs are few and often unreliable. The body may show signs of maceration, indicating that death occurred within the uterus, or there may be some gross congenital abnormality, such that a child could not live. An examination of the umbilical cord may assist. It begins to shrivel within 12 to 24 hours after delivery, but changes in the cord between delivery and 12 hours or so can only be seen on microscopic examination. A still-birth umbilicus shows none of the changes.

The main part of the internal examination is devoted to the lungs, and in particular to their buoyancy when placed in water. It is termed the 'hydrostatic test'. It may seem crude and almost non-scientific because of its simplicity. If, when the lungs are placed in water, they sink, they are lungs that have no inspired air, and therefore they are the lungs from a stillbirth. If, on the other hand, they float freely, it indicates that the child has breathed before it died, and therefore had a separate existence.

The author, on occasions, has found that separating the lungs or even parts of a lung before placing them in water, as proposed by some experts has produced spurious results. Are they sinking or floating?

In my view, the best way is to remove the entire neck and thoracic organs together, and place the entire specimen in the water. The lungs if they really contain air will be able to support the weight of the remaining organs. If the lungs are undubitably airless or there is uncertainty, then the structures will all sink.

Two possible complications must not be overlooked when applying the test. First, the possibility of putrefaction of all the tissues, including the lungs, with the formation of gas bubbles. These are formed in the tissues by certain strains of bacteria. It may be alleged that the gas bubbles will assist the lungs to float. However the absence of putrefraction anywhere else in the body will help to prevent any misconception or misunderstanding. The second problem may arise, if it is thought that there may have been some attempt at artificial respiration, especially the mouth-to-mouth technique. It is generally considered doubtful whether this method is really effective in instituting normal breathing where none has previously existed.

To exclude extraneous, non-intra-alveolar gas or air bubbles external pressure should be applied to the lungs before performing the hydrostatic test. The author has found that by placing the lungs between two layers of cloth and applying firm pressure with the foot, the excess pressure will force out any gases from the major air passages, yet, surprisingly this procedure does not affect the state of the alveoli. If they have been previously expanded by normal respiration they will return to that state; and will float when returned to the water. To confirm these opinions, representative pieces of the lungs should be sent to the laboratory for microscopical examination.

Should the hydrostatic test be equivocal and microscopy also prove unhelpful then the decision is made that the child has not had a separate existence.

Additional tests, although less important, are designed to determine whether air is present in the stomach and upper intestine but sometimes the results are unhelpful.

Time of death

Bodies are sometimes found on waste ground, in dustbins or blocked in waste water pipes, and the investigating team frequently and quite properly asks when the infant died. Coupled with this question is the matter of age at death. In many cases there is no question of a separate existence; the infant has lived for some time, perhaps a day or two, and then been destroyed. Probably the only help that can be obtained from the body itself is from the umbilical stump. By the end of the second day a clearly defined red reaction surrounds the stump, and by the third or fourth day there are signs of separation. The stump is cast off by the end of the first week.

The timing of death is extremely difficult to ascertain. Often the body is discarded so that the taking of any temperature readings is valueless. Even rigor mortis is so poor as to be almost undetectable. Generally speaking very little help can be given in this regard.

Natural death

Natural death in the first 60 to 72 hours of life is of importance because it is in this time that child murder is most likely. Many of the natural deaths occur in premature babies – a premature baby is defined as one with a birth weight of less than 5½lb. Other causes include congenital abnormalities, mainly of the cardiovascular system. Severe congenital heart or lung disease is amenable to surgery, but only if recognized early enough.

Biochemical disorders and metabolic diseases may cause an early death, but usually not in the immediate post-natal period.

Severe cerebral disorders or defects of the spinal canal and cord, if they do not result in stillbirth, may cause death in the early post-natal period. A well-known example is 'spina-bifida' with its several complications. After the immediate post-natal period,

275

many infant deaths are the result of infection, usually when the ante-natal and post-natal care and attention could be described as totally inadequate.

Inattention at birth

Often a new-born infant is found dead in suspicious circumstances without any marks of violence on the body. It appears to have been just abandoned. Having determined that the infant had had a separate existence, the question of 'causing its death by omitting to take due care' arises.

The conclusion that the infant died from lack of attention is drawn from a number of factors. First of these is the site of the discovery of the body – in a dustbin, on open ground etc. – there appear to be attempts to dispose of it illegally. Second is the absence of any normal attention to the infant – the umbilical cord has not been properly separated and ligated, the infant has not been washed. Third, there appear to have been no formal preparations for its arrival – no clothing, no bedding and no special baby materials. In summary, there is a general air of abandonment at the place where the baby was born.

Nevertheless the conclusion can only be drawn once the autopsy has been completed, in order to exclude any natural disease which could have contributed to or caused the death.

Act of commission

There is almost no limit to the methods by which the new-born infant can be destroyed, even by an exhausted and perhaps a frightened and inexperienced mother. The infant can be smothered by a cushion or a pillow, leaving behind little or no evidence of the fact on the face, which in itself is difficult to distinguish from a natural death. The child can be strangled either manually or by a ligature. One form of ligature close at hand is the umbilical cord. But it has to be admitted that sometimes a baby is born with the umbilical cord entangled around its neck.

Deliberate violence is sometimes used by striking the child's head against the floor or the wall causing severe brain damage. Again the problem of natural brain haemorrhage following a difficult delivery may arise, and a precipitate unexpected delivery whilst standing might be said to cause the skull fracture as the baby fell to the floor. Drowning the child is often used. The child is placed in the toilet pan or in the bath, but the story given is again a precipitate delivery whilst the mother was sitting on the toilet or taking a bath or shower. Instrumental death however is more obvious. Stabbing by means of a knife or scissors produces fairly characteristic wounds to the body. However as the illustration below suggests, there may be an innocent explanation.

Example   A new-born infant was found on the floor of a toilet in a house. The mother was in the house and was hysterical and gave no coherent story. The child's body had numerous, widely spaced, stab wounds in bizarre places. What at first looked like a frenzied homicide was shown later to have been the result of multiple blows by a toilet brush. The woman had been all alone in the house and had delivered the baby whilst sitting on the toilet. She had fainted away from blood loss.

277

Meanwhile the baby's head was all the time under the water and it drowned. In her distraught state, after she discovered what had happened, the mother used the handle with a pronounced point to it, to try to flush the baby away round the bend of the toilet. Thus the wounds were post mortem wounds.

SUDDEN INFANT DEATH SYNDROME

THE syndrome ('SIDS') is more often referred to by the general public as 'cot death', and today it is the most common cause of infant mortality after the perinatal period. The annual number of cot deaths now exceeds the combined numbers for deaths from congenital diseases, malignant diseases and accidents.

Throughout the whole of Western Europe and from other study centres around the world, the average rate is about one death for every 500 live births. This means that in the UK alone about 1200–1500 deaths occur each year from cot death. Over the past 30 years improved community health care has lowered steadily the total infant mortality, but SIDS deaths has remained largely unchanged. The result is that SIDS deaths are now much more prominent than previously.

Cases of cot deaths may occur between the ages of two weeks and two years, but the majority of cases occur between two and seven months, the main incidence being around three months. Most surveys reveal a slight increase in the number of male deaths, but this is a fact seen in most diseases throughout life. There is a definite increased risk when there are twins, as opposed to single babies. The increase is said to be three to five times higher but no reasonable explanation has been yet forthcoming.

Cot deaths have an association with the season. They are almost restricted to the colder months in both the northern and southern hemispheres. In warmer climates such as the tropics the incidence of SIDS deaths is low by comparison with temperate zones, but is evenly spread throughout the year.

Perhaps the most remarkable feature about deaths due to SIDS is the time of day at which death occurs. Almost all the deaths occur during sleep and in the early hours of the morning, between 2am and 6am. A small group die between 2pm and 6pm and an even smaller group die late in the morning or in the evening.

Cot deaths can occur in any family, and many cases have occurred in families of the more privileged classes, although the majority of cases do appear in families in the lower socio-economic groups.

Example   A three-month old baby was unwell during the day with very mild respiratory systems, but not sufficiently distressing for the mother to seek medical or nursing help. He received a normal 10pm bottle feed but was restless and 'grizzly'. Mother gave him some boiled water at 12 midnight and a further small feed at 2am, after which he settled and slept. At the time of his early morning feed (around 5.30am) he was found dead in his cot. There had been no vomiting, sweating or movement in his cot.

The post mortem findings are essentially negative. There are no abnormal external findings and internally the findings in the thorax are non-specific. Classic cases will show scattered petechial (pinpoint)

279

haemorrhages on and in the thymus, on the posterior surface of the heart and on the pleural surfaces of the lower lobes of the lungs. The lungs show 'geographical' areas of pink and purple on the surface and on serial slicing, these represent normal and congestive areas, and nothing else. Although these signs suggest a mechanical asphyxia, there is no evidence to support this theory.

The explanatory theories are numerous. They range from a wide selection of viruses, to hypothermia, allergy to cow's milk and abnormal nervous conducting systems in the heart.

Until the cause is known, there are no preventative measures that can be put forward, apart from intense supervision of high-risk children, which for most families is impractical.

There is, however, a real need for comfort and supportive counselling to the bereaved parents, and many children's hospitals have cot death support groups. Whilst all professional workers who have contact with a cot death tragedy must not instigate a 'witch-hunt', it has to be said that a post mortem examination of the body is essential in every case to exclude the possibility of an unlawful killing.

NON-ACCIDENTAL INJURY IN CHILDHOOD

THIS state or condition is also referred to as 'the battered baby' or 'battered child syndrome' or simply as child abuse. Perhaps the original term should be extended to 'repetitive non-accidental injury in childhood' to highlight that the abuse and cruelty is not from an isolated fit of rage but from deliberate acts committed time and again.

The child is usually under the age of two years, although some cases are seen up to four years. Undoubtedly more subtle forms of abuse including sexual abuse occur up to puberty and even later.

The family, often an unmarried mother living with the father, or the mother living with the non-biological father, is often seen as being maladjusted, immature and under continual stress. The injuries and the explanation offered by the parents do not agree. The explanations are readily offered with over-protective attitude by the parents. On the other hand there is often an inexplicable delay between the onset of the injuries and the time that medical help is sought. The child is usually taken to the hospital rather than the family doctor. It may be that there is the chance that the child will be examined each time by a different, unsuspecting doctor.

The child is usually, but not invariably, the only child to be assaulted, and it is done out of view of the other, older children. They are told 'Johnny has been naughty again!' Often the abused child is a premature child. One's natural inclination is to assume that the normal 'maternal instinct' would engender more, not less, affection for the child. The premature child may be backward in the normal 'milestones' in life, e.g. sitting up, feeding itself, toilet training. The continual slowness or backwardness generates frustration and tension and the feelings are released in abusive acts.

All social classes may assault their children, cases having been prosecuted amongst professional and educated parents, but most cases are found in the lower socio-economic groups.

Clinical examination

On examination abrasions and bruises are found in many places on the body, even the places inaccessible to normal falling or bumping against objects. The bruises are usually of different ages, indicative of repetition. There may be injuries to the lips and mouth, especially to the inside of the lips or gums with possible displacement or dislodgement of some teeth. Burns from many souces, especially cigarette burns, are frequently seen, or circular scars from previous burns. More serious injuries include multiple fractures, mainly to the skull and the long bones of the limbs. A full X-ray is indicated to determine not only the full extent of the skeletal damage, but also to assess the ages of the fractures, whether recent or in varying stages of repair. Injuries to the eyes, especially retinal haemorrhages from vigorous shaking of the head, are fairly common. There may be bite marks on the soft fatty areas such as shoulders, arms, buttocks and thighs.

Bizarre sadistic injuries are sometimes seen following scalding, beating, sexual interference and even incised wounds.

It has been estimated that for a child examined for bodily inuuries inflicted by a parent there is a 60 per cent chance of returning to the doctor with a recurrence of injuries at a later date and at least 10 per cent possibility that the child will eventually die from further injuries.

Pathological findings

Cerebral haemorrhages, both extracerebral and intracerebral, may be found, either from violent shaking of the head, or direct blows to the top or side of the head. Haemorrhages may also be found in the abdominal cavity following lacerations to the liver, spleen, mesentary and even the intestines. Microscopical evidence of former peritoneal infection or previous haemorrhage may be seen.

These findings will provide an adequate cause of death

The role of the professional

It should not be forgotten that this syndrome is not new. Many of the nineteenth century novels contain direct or oblique references to child abuse. However it was forgotten or overlooked and in 1946 Caffey first described a case of subdural haemorrhage in association with fractured limb bones. In 1957 he suggested parental neglect as a cause for the finding. Then in 1962 Kempe et al attributed child injuries to deliberate parental assaults, coining the term 'battered baby syndrome'. It was met with considerable incredulity by many of the medical practitioners, who sought disease processes to explain the findings. Thus many cases were missed until the realization of what was happening in society eventually dawned on them.

Today, many agencies are actively engaged in the work of protecting the child at risk. Local health authorities have created 'at-risk' registers on which all the details of known or suspected children are entered. Thereafter the case committee of the social services department can regularly sit and review the case and can arrange regular house visits to supervise the situation.

Many professionals interact in the welfare of these children-at-risk. General practitioners, district nurses, the societies for the prevention of cruelty to children, health visitors, churches and other voluntary agencies all have a part to play.

Regrettably, finding an acceptable solution to this insidious social evil is less easy than it seems, and time and again the system breaks down and there are failures which have led to the death of a child. Naturally the news media view such repeated failures as scandalous.

At the moment, the system of advice, help and supervision is directed to the innocent child, and this is right and proper, but the parents, too, are in need of help.

It must be incumbent on society to help inadequate parents or unstable families in stressful situations. For them the circumstances are often so hopeless that the only outlet for frustration is on the weakest member of the family.

Whilst cases of serious assault, especially when it is to the endangerment of life, cannot be allowed to go untried and unpunished, very often that is too late – the child is then maimed or even dead. All professional and expert help must be utilized at an early stage by society to prevent such tragedies; otherwise it might be again too late.

REFERENCES

Caffey, J. (1946), *Am. J. Roentg.,* **56**,163.
Caffey, J. (1957), *Br. J. Radiol.*, **30**, 225.
Kempe, C.H., Silverman, F.N., Steele, B.F., Droegmueller, W. & Silver, H.K. (1962), *J.Am.-Med.Assoc.*, **181**,17.

13   SEXUAL OFFENCES

It is a popular misconception that forensic medicine is concerned only with post mortem examinations. Nevertheless it is true that the medical evidence presented in court tends to be heavily weighted towards describing in detail the various wounds and injuries found on a corpse. But forensic medicine also includes the clinical examination of living subjects, and victims of sexual offences form a large part of the clinical work. Usually such intimate examinations are performed by a police surgeon, or a general practitioner called in to assist in particular examinations, rather than a forensic pathologist, but at times both may become involved. Thus the examination of victims of sexual offences is an example of clinical and pathological cooperation.

GENERAL LEGAL CONSIDERATIONS

Before we begin to consider the general clinical examination and then the specific genital examination, it would be helpful to look at the general legal principles which govern the various sexual offences.

Rape

Rape is the most serious of the sexual offences and is defined as 'unlawful sexual intercourse by a man with a woman who, at the time of intercourse, does not consent, or is reckless as to whether she consents' (Sexual Offences (Amendment) Act 1976). This definition is statutorily applied in England and Wales, for, in Scotland, rape is a crime at common law, defined as 'the carnal knowledge of a female by a male person obtained by overcoming her will'. The merest penetration of the penis between the labia against her consent is sufficient to constitute the offence.

The lack of consent may also be due to the fact that the female is technically or legally unable to grant a valid consent. She may be suffering from severe mental abnormality or disease within the terms of the Mental Health Acts and therefore she is not in a position to make a considered judgement, or she may be under the age of 16 years, the age of consent. The woman may be unable to grant consent because she has been subjugated by force, fear or fraud, or as the result of some intoxicating or stupefying drugs.

Intercourse with a girl under 16 years

Special considerations have been given in the UK to acts of sexual intercourse with girls below the age of 16 years and above the age of 13 years in England, or 12 years in Scotland. Where there has been no overt objection to the act, or to the attempt to carry out the act, the offence is described as having, or attempting to have sexual intercourse, rather than as rape. In most of the cases considered under this heading, not only has there been no objection, but a willing cooperation by the young girl. The cases therefore are regarded as being less serious than those of the offence of rape. There is a statutory defence open to the male offender, if he can show that at the time of the offence he was under the age of 24 years, that he had not been charged previously with a similar offence, that he had no knowledge that the girl was under 16 years, and that he had reasonable cause (from her dress, build, appearance etc.) to believe that she was older than 16 years.

In all cases of the under 16-year-old girls who have objected, or where fear, force, fraud or stupefying drugs have been used, the offence is then considered to be rape.

Indecent assault

Any unlawful sexual contact that falls short of rape or attempted rape, because there is no actual or attempted penile penetration, is termed indecent assault. The essential point in the offence is the lack of consent by the victim. Consent is not valid, even if given, if the female is under the age of 16 years, or if she is suffering from mental abnormality or disease or is under the influence of drugs or the consent has been invalidly granted by reason of force, fear or fraud. There is no subdivision into girls above and below the age of 13 years in England, or 12 years in Scotland as is the case with sexual intercourse.

Indecent assault may vary from the merest touching of thighs or breasts to handling and digital penetration of the vagina or anus or oro-genital contact. An actual assault must have taken place in order to establish a charge of indecent assault, but where there has not been an assault, charges under the Indecency with Children Act, 1960 can be brought. In Scotland, such cases are brought under common law when the child is below the age of 12, and are termed 'lewd and libidinous practices'. Between the ages of 12 and 16 the offence is dealt with under the Sexual Offences (Scotland) Act 1976.

Incest

Although there are some differences between Scots law and the law applied in England and Wales, in general terms the offence is that of a man having intercourse with his mother, sister, daughter, granddaughter or half-sister, aunt or niece. The same degree of relationship are prohibited between a woman and her male relatives of similar degrees of consanguinity. Recent changes in Scots law involve parents and adopted children and also between persons in guardianship, trust or in authority and the subject of that special relationship. Apart from the actual offence of incest, there may also be an offence by virtue of the girl being under the age of 16 years. The conditions for proving that incest has occurred are the practial ones as for rape, namely, that there has been vulval penetration. Unfortunately cases rarely come to be reported until after the offence has been practised for some time and then only when there is a pregnancy, or some sexually transmitted disease present or there is a family break-up because of what has occurred.

Homosexual offences

Between consenting women, an offence is not committed, unless one of them is under the age of 16 years and is thereby unable to consent to what is then termed an indecent assault. In certain circumstances, even between consenting adult women, a charge of gross indecency could be brought.

Between men, the laws of both England and Scotland are now in general agreement. Acts of anal intercourse are no longer criminal offences provided that the acts are performed between consenting males, who have attained the age of 21 years and that they are performed in private. It is, nevertheless, a criminal offence if one of the men is under 21 years, despite the age of majority being 18 years, or if practised between Merchant Navy seamen on board ship, or between members of the armed services or if one of the partners is female. The term 'private place' is strictly interpreted. It excludes public places such as public toilets, a frequent place for homosexual activities. To substantiate a charge under the Sexual Offences Acts, the proof of penetration by the penis of the anus suffices; the proof of seminal emission is unnecessary.

MEDICAL EXAMINATION

THE following preliminary procedures must be adhered to.

For whom is the examination to be conducted

It is of the utmost importance that, at the outset, all

who have any interest in the examination are made aware as to who has requested the examination and therefore is entitled to receive the subsequent report of the medical findings. In an emotionally charged atmosphere, with instructions coming from several directions, the doctor must be sure that he has the full approval of the police officer in charge of the case, the procurator fiscal, or some other legal authority, and it is courteous to notify the victim's personal doctor, with her consent, in case there is a need for follow-up medical attention.

The full details of the person to be examined

The identity of the victim must be established and full personal details duly recorded before the examination commences.

The place of examination

It will be of importance in any future court proceedings to record the time, date and place of the examination as well as the names of those present at the time. The time interval between the alleged assault and the examination should be recorded.

Consent to the examination

At the outset of the interview the informed consent of the victim must be obtained by the doctor or, in the case of a child, from the parent or guardian both for the medical examination and for the publishing of his subsequent report. From the victim herself oral consent is sufficient, if given before a witness but in the case of a minor, or a female suffering from mental disability, the responsible adult should commit her consent to writing. No consent should be accepted until the consenting party has had a full explanation of what exactly is proposed to be done.

A short medical history

A general medical history should be outlined, but should include details of past illnesses, accidents and surgical operations. It should also include details of any recent illness and, in particular, any treatment given for the illness. Along with details of medicines, the victim should be asked details of any alcohol consumption during the 24 hours before the alleged offence.

A gynaecological and, where appropriate, an obstetric history should be obtained and recorded. This must include the date of the last menstrual period and the use of any contraceptive medication or appliances. The obstetric history is designed to discover whether any vaginal or vulval injury may have occurred during delivery which then required surgery.

Sexual history

Remembering that serious allegations have been made, it is necessary to inquire discreetly but without timidity into past sexual experience. This should be directed along two lines: first, whether the female is claiming to have been a virgin before the assault took place, and second, if virginity is not in question, then the inquiry should be directed towards all acts of intercourse engaged in, with her consent, during the preceding two weeks or since the last menstrual period if this is sooner. This line of questioning is of considerable relevance if the alleged victim is a woman who is cohabiting regularly with her partner. It is of importance in the later study of the seminal fluid and spermatozoa by the scientists.

Specific history of the alleged offence

This may prove difficult to obtain, especially if the victim is in shock, or suffering from revulsion, horror and any physical pain caused by the attack. Specific questions should not be avoided, such as the time of the attack, the place and the circumstances and whether the complaint was made soon afterwards or delayed for some reason.

Some idea of the degree of force can be obtained by asking the patient whether she was restrained in some way whether her clothes were torn off her or forcibly removed and whether she put up any resistance.

Additional questions should be put concerning the details of the act, whether it was a single episode or repeated, whether ejaculation occurred to her knowledge and whether any abnormal sexual acts also occurred.

Finally the victim must be asked whether she has washed herself or any part of her body since the incident occurred, or changed any of her clothes, and if so what has become of them.

THE CLINICAL EXAMINATION

A complete clinical examination is required in every case, and must therefore include such details as the person's weight, height and general build, in particular a comment on muscular development and probable power to resist an assault. A note should be made of the patient's general demeanour, her understanding of the situation and her attitude to the examination.

Is there evidence of residual shock, fear, resentment or disgust or any trace of worry concerning possible future consequencs? These are all important features that must be included in the report and which may have a significant bearing at any future legal proceedings.

Whilst it will be necessary for the victim to undress completely to allow for a detailed clinical examination, a suitable loose-fitting gown should be provided for warmth and modesty. It must never be forgotten that there will be a natural reluctance on the part of a woman, and even more so in the case of a girl, to undress in front of a male doctor, bearing in mind the preceding distressful events. Therefore the services of a female attendant must be on hand. Whilst a close relative or friend of the victim is very useful, a woman police officer should also be there to observe the actual undressing process, so that she can report anything of relevance to the doctor. It is now standard practice for the victim to stand on a large sheet of brown paper whilst undressing so that any contact traces dropping from the clothes, for example, hairs, fibres, vegetation, can be collected up and sent for a scientific examination.

Collection of clothing

Many police forces supply examination rooms with
boxed kits for the medical and scientific investigation
of alleged sexual offences. These contain large sheets
of brown paper, swabs, microscope slides, syringes
and needles, tubes for blood and saliva collections, a
comb, and an assortment of bags, envelopes and
labels.

If it is considered necessary for the clothing to be
removed for a scientific investigation at the laboratory, then the alleged victim or her companion should
be asked to bring along another set of clothing in
which to return home.

Each item of clothing should be identified and
labelled and placed in a separate clean brown paper
bag. Plastic bags should not be used as they retain any
moisture present and this will encourage the growth
of moulds on the clothing, as well as retaining any
unpleasant smells.

EXTERNAL EXAMINATION

Head and neck

Beginning at the top of the head, palpation is made
for painful or sore areas caused by blows and giving
rise to abrasions or bruises. The search continues
over the back of the neck and around the ears where
'rabbit-chops' are sometimes given. Next examine
the eyes and eyelids for any petechial haemorrhages;
their presence may support a claim of attempted
strangulation. The nostrils may contain some blood

from a blow. The lips should be examined on both the outer and inner surfaces for bruises or small lacerations. These may have been caused by violent attempts at kissing, or by the knuckles of a hand, either delivering a blow to the face, or more likely, the pressure of a hand on the mouth to prevent screaming.

Apart from attempts at strangulation, which may produce a number of indistinct bruises on the front and sides of the neck, there may be one or more circular bruises on the side of the neck, the so-called 'love bites' which are not true bite marks but are caused by sucking the skin very hard.

Trunk

The area of back, chest and abdomen require special attention, because although the victim may complain of stiffness, soreness and vague pains, the external signs are often quite difficult to see. Bruising of the breasts and over the scapular regions are the most frequently found signs, but even then, they are often indistinct. The former bruises are caused by rough handling or squeezing with maximal tenderness round the nipples, whilst the latter are caused by the back wriggling in resistance, against a hard and perhaps roughened surface. The breasts should also be examined for bite marks and perhaps love bites. Bite marks leave behind an impact abrasion in a roughly oval shape, caused by the biting edges of the incisor and canine teeth. Often there is localized bruising in association with the pit depressions caused by each tooth.

A forensic odontologist will probably be able to

prepare swabs from the bite marks made on the skin and then he will try to prepare a plaster or plastic impression of the entire bitten area for comparative and evidential purposes at a later date.

It is essential that the forensic odontologist or a dental surgeon be alerted to the presence of a bite mark as soon as possible, if he is to get any information at all from the mark.

The limbs

It is important to examine each limb from all sides. Using a self-devised systematic scheme, in order not to leave any part of the skin unexamined, search and record any bruises, abrasions, minor lacerations, soiling, blood and broken nails. Such information may provide valuable evidence in determining the nature of the attack and whether any resistance by the victim was at all possible. Finger-tip bruising on the arms consistent with gripping are occasionally seen around the wrists, forearms and also on the inner aspect of the thighs. This last site may show a larger more diffuse area of bruising caused by the legs being forced apart by pressure from the thighs of the assailant.

If the fingernails are long enough, and there is reason to suspect that the assailant has been scratched by the victim, a collection of the victim's nail scrapings may prove of value.

EXAMINATION OF THE GENITALIA

IT cannot be overstressed that this examination must

be conducted in a good light, with the woman lying on her back, in the so-called lithotomy position, on a firm examination couch with ample opportunity for the doctor to move easily all round it. Sufficient time must be allowed for the doctor to make a careful systematic examination of each part separately.

In the case of young children, a great deal of patience and gentleness are necessary before gaining the confidence of the child to allow you to separate the legs and handle the genitalia. Small incentives such as a new toy or a few sweets often have miraculous powers in an otherwise difficult situation.

The examination begins with the pubic hair in order to see whether there be matted seminal or foreign material present. Suspicious areas should be carefully cut away and preserved. This may now be followed by a careful combing of the pubic hair as dissimilar male hairs may be present. A cut sample of the woman's pubic hair must be taken for comparison.

The vulva is next examined beginning with the clitoris and proceeding to look at each of the labia majora and minora, followed by an inspection of the urethral opening ending finally at the fourchette, behind the vagina, and the perineum. The entire area will be checked for abrasions, probably presenting as minor scratches, such as might be caused by fingernails, any bruising, reddening or tender swelling. In the case of a child, thought must be given to the possibility that areas of reddening with fine scratch marks might be due to poor vulval hygiene, resulting in irritation by urine etc.

Attention is then turned to the vagina. To begin with, hymenal, low vaginal and high vaginal swabs together with the aspiration of any vaginal fluid by means of a pipette must always be performed before any digital or instrumental exploration can be conducted. The possibility that semen deposited on the vulva away from the vagina being carried in accidentally by the fingers or instruments can therefore be discounted if the swabs and aspiration are always made the first steps in the vaginal examination. From the swabs, smear preparations can be made on the microscope slides and the material immediately 'fixed' on to the slide by means of a preparatory cytological wax/acetone/ether fixative. It enables the smears to be 'protected' during transport to the laboratory.

The hymen should next be inspected and the presence of any recent hymenal injury noted. Considerable experience is required by the examining doctor before making some decisions, because the anatomy of the hymen varies so much from one individual to another. It may be thin and elastic and almost translucent, or it may be thick, rather rigid, opaque, and resistant to finger pressure. The opening in the hymen can vary a lot from a crescentic slit, to a large orifice with a markedly crenated border. Sometimes the hymen is deficient anteriorly and thicker than average posteriorly.

Because of the anatomical direction of the vagina, the maximal damage to the hymen on the first penetration is to the posterior portion. It is there that recent tears will be readily seen. However, if the hymen is elastic it may stretch considerably before any tears appear and the degree of rupture is thereby lessened, and may be surprisingly small. When the hymen ruptures, the tear or tears will extend back to the firm vaginal wall, being the margin of the hymen. It is widely held that finger or tampon insertion may cause only partial tearing, thus still preserving virginity, whilst penile penetration will complete the tear to reach the vaginal wall. There must be exceptions to these views and it all depends on so many factors, such as frequency of insertion, the size of the respective parts, the degree of force, the use of lubricants and the speed or otherwise of insertion.

As a working general rule, bearing in mind these factors, if any small tears are present and they do not extend to the vaginal wall, then the female should be considered as still virgo intacta.

Sometimes in the absence of hymenal rupture, attempts at penetration by a penis or other object will produce an abrasion at the vaginal orifice and an area of bruising on the hymen. These should be carefully looked for and recorded.

On occasions tearing of the hymen by forceful penile penetration can produce tissue damage at a much further distance in the vagina. There may be an abrasion or actual vaginal tearing on the posterior wall, and in order to see this it will be necessary to insert a suitably sized speculum, but great care and patience is required to insert it. In the case of very young children it will probably require a general anaesthetic before it can be achieved.

One method of examining the hymen is to carefully insert one of a series of Glaister Keen glass rods. Each consists of a glass rod on the end of which there is a glass sphere of increasing size. The more elaborate ones are internally illuminated. The appropriate sized sphere is passed through the hymenal orifice and moved about so that the edge of the hymen is spread over the illuminated area. This will allow any small recent tear to be clearly seen with the light coming from behind the hymen.

The vaginal examination ends by a deep vaginal examination, if this can be tolerated by the patient, as occasionally high vaginal tears have been known to occur after violent assaults, especially in the smaller younger persons.

Finally, a venous sample and a saliva sample are obtained for blood grouping and secretor status and together with the vaginal swabs, vaginal aspirate and microscope slide preparations are all sent to the laboratory.

The entire investigation of a rape case including the history taking and the questioning of the alleged victim must be undertaken with thought, care and, above all, with the highest standards of professionalism.

Recent campaigning by women's action groups against certain methods of police investigation into alleged sexual offeces, and against male doctors undertaking the intimate examinations, demands that all professional persons involved in a case demonstrate a high degree of integrity and objectivity. However they must also show understanding and reasonableness in these unfortunate and tragic cases.

EXAMINATION OF THE SUSPECTED ASSAILANT

IT is much more the case that the victim of a sexual assault will be brought to the doctor to be examined than the assailant. The problem for the doctor regarding the assailant is that if and when he is apprehended and brought to the doctor, there is usually an inordinate delay which may range from a number of hours up to several days later. Such a delay makes it difficult to conduct an external examination and to evaluate any findings.

The procedure begins as in the case of the victim by explaining clearly what is to happen, recording carefully all his personal data and taking great pains to obtain his consent before proceeding further. The man should be asked if he is wearing the same clothes as at the time of the alleged assault, and if he is prepared to release them for a scientific investigation.

As in the case of the female, the medical examination concentrates on two separate areas. There is first the general body examination, looking for and recording any fingernail abrasions on the face, neck, back, buttocks and arms. If any are present, it is in order to ask him for an explanation of how they occurred, if he is able to do so. The body is also inspected for any signs of mud, soil, blood or vegetable material. Clearly, the longer the delay in examining the man, the less chance of finding anything unusual.

The second area of inspection is the genital region. If this is examined shortly after the alleged assault, there may be signs of swelling, tenderness and minor degrees of reddening or bruising around the base of the glans penis and on the frenulum. Although when seen the penis will be soft and flaccid, a note of the possible penile size when erect is useful especially in relation to any damage on the female. Samples of pubic hair should be removed for the purposes of comparison, and any matted areas should also be carefully cut away. The scrotum and testes should also be examined for any pathological findings.

As in the case of the female, samples of venous blood and saliva should be collected for blood group-

ing and secretor status determination. If the delay
between the offences and the examination is unduly
long, many of these details can be omitted.

EXAMINATION IN CASES OF ANAL INTERCOURSE

A medical examination of both the passive and active
partners will probably be asked for, where an alleged
act of anal intercourse has occurred outside of the
terms of the Sexual Offences Acts, in which specific
conditions are laid down.

As in the case of alleged heterosexual sexual offences, before any kind of examination can take place,
the precise reasons for it must be fully explained and
the person's informed consent obtained.

It is necessary to begin by taking a general medical
history from the victim or, where appropriate, the
passive partner, or if too young to understand, from
the parent or guardian. The questioning will be specially directed to the bowel habits, including previous
constipation, or diarrhoea, and irritation, the presence of haemorrhoids, and whether any form of local treatment has been applied, including the use of
suppositories. It is prudent to ask whether at any
previous time, acts of anal intercourse have ever
taken place, and to record any details of the circumstances given.

A general external examination of the undressed
body will precede a more detailed examination of the
anus and its surroundings. The general examination
will be directed towards any abrasions from fingernails, or from instruments and objects of bondage
and restraint, or from contact with roughened objects

and surfaces such as furniture or the floor on which the victim was held down.

Other important points include the presence and site of any bruises, swelling and skin contamination with soil, blood, faeces, semen or vegetable matter. Where appropriate the clothing worn at the time of the alleged incident should be retained and sent to the forensic scientists for a detailed study.

An examination of the anal area and the genitalia will follow. Before any finger contact by the examiner is made, swabs from the anal verge, the skin of the perineum and from just within the anal canal, must be taken. These will be examined both for traces of semen and for lubricating substances.

Around the anus there may be tissue swelling, bruising, tenderness, bleeding skin tags, some faecal soiling and the tendency for the sphincter of the anus to be in spasm, because of pain. These signs are usually seen in a first-time anal intercourse, when forcibly undertaken and in young males.

Different features are found in the case of a willing and experienced passive partner. The normal folds at the anal margin tend to be absent, giving to the margin a smooth appearance. There may be a number of small distinct white or pinkish linear scars from healed former fissures. In extreme cases of habituation to anal intercourse, the anus appears to be 'funnelled', with the actual anal opening deeply set in the funnel.

For pathologists, used to examining the anus in a cadaver, they have to remember that the anus in life is normally in a closed slit-like state, and it will exert a natural firm spasmic grip on the examining finger, so that comments on the degree of 'grip' in examining a victim must be tempered with caution.

The examination of the active partner, or the assailant, in anal intercourse follows the same difficult path as for the assailant in a case of forced vaginal intercourse. He is rarely examined soon after the event, thus giving him a greater opportunity for washing the genital organs and changing his clothes. Nevertheless, even in late medical examinations, possible contact between the two parties can still be determined through studies on pubic hair, blood, saliva and possibly semen. In an examination undertaken shortly after the act, minor injuries may be detected at the base of the glans penis, as well as finding traces of lubricant or faecal soiling on the shaft of the penis or even in the pubic hair. As with the victim, the clothing should be removed for examination, where special attention will be paid to the crutch or front of the underpants or the fly or crutch of the trousers, for semen, lubricant or faecal material.

14   DROWNING

To a non-professional, death by drowning is due to the apparently simple process of obstructing the air passages with water. In fact, it is a far more complicated process both pathologically and biochemically. The picture is further confused by the wide range of appearances that may be presented to the pathologist, ranging from the near-normal to the full classical signs both externally and on dissection. The truth of the matter is that to diagnose death by drowning is one of the hardest tasks in forensic medicine.

Whenever a body is recovered dead from the water several questions present themselves. These are:

1   Was the person alive when he entered the water?

2   If he was alive why could he not save himself?

3   If he was alive did he die from drowning or from sudden immersion in water?

4   If he was already dead when he entered the water, from what did he die?

5   Were any injuries found on the body caused

before entry, during his entry, or as a result of being in the water?

6   When did he enter the water, in terms of hours, days or weeks?

In seeking answers we need to consider

  (a)   his situation before entry,
  (b)   his condition on entry, and
  (c)   the events that followed until his recovery.

Before entry

It must be established whether the victim was alive before he entered the water. Such enquiries will centre on his mental state, in particular, whether he had ever discussed, or even attempted suicide and for what reasons. When was he last seen alive?

Perhaps the man was suffering from some chronic physical disease such as ischaemic heart disease or high blood pressure, and this precipitated a full blown heart attack, and he simply fell into the water during the attack.

An alternative situation might be that it was a pure accident such as losing his grip, or balance, whilst walking or working near water.

Rarely, but dramatically, he might have received a blow to the head, rendering him unconscious and was then pushed into the water, as part of a criminal act.

All of these examples presume him to be alive when he entered the water and death could therefore be either from drowning or from immersion.

DROWNING

On entry

The views of any onlookers will prove to be of considerable value, because they could describe whether there was a desperate struggle for survival, or whether he suddenly disappeared. The first scenario would be more likely to produce the classical findings of drowning in the body whilst the second may show nothing at all.

Injuries to the body may be found following contact with any object prior to entering the water, or possibly due to striking rocks, or the bottom of a shallow pool, after entry. The site and appearance of the wounds could be of some value in understanding his death.

Recovery

Even if a person is observed falling into water such as a river, loch or the sea, it may take some time, perhaps several days or occasionally weeks, to recover the body. Post mortem changes can often be very marked in the form of skin changes, decomposition, post mortem mutilation and, covered by silt and mud, identification of the body is often very difficult to establish. It often takes a full autopsy with dental studies to be certain of a person's identity even after a period of two or three weeks.

POST MORTEM EXAMINATION

IN a body *recently* recovered from the water there may be a marked 'goose-skin' appearance to the entire skin, and a curious white, soggy, crinkled appearance to the skin of the hands and feet – 'washerwoman's hands'.

Froth, in the form of a fine white or pink-tinged texture may be seen at the nose and mouth, or if not present, it can often be made to appear after applying pressure to the front of the chest. A record must be made of any injuries present, in the light of what was said above about ante-mortem injuries.

On opening the chest, the unmistakable feature of drowning will be seen, when the large, ballooned or hyperinflated lungs will almost escape from the thorax. Each lobe shows pronounced sharp borders as each part, previously unexpanded, is now filled to the limit.

The froth may be seen to extend down the trachea and perhaps well into the bronchi. There may also be excess free fluid present, but not down into the very small branches which together with the surrounding lung tissue appear remarkably dry. The water has pushed and compressed the air in front of it to the limits of the air passages. Other findings may include excess fluid in the stomach with perhaps some foreign matter such as vegetation or silt. (On one notable occasion the author discovered a small intact fish in the stomach!)

A recent finding, and one worthy of further study, is the presence of haemorrhages in the air spaces of the middle ear and mastoid air cells caused by unequal hydrostatic and barometric pressures in the ears. It is a very strong indication that death was caused by drowning. It is rarely seen in other forms of asphyxial death.

Mention must be made of the tests for diatoms. The presence of these acid-resistant silica shells of certain plankton in such sites as the liver, bone marrow and brain are useful markers that death was due to drowning. It is believed that they enter the lungs with the water, pass into the circulation and are deposited or trapped by these organs. They are useful markers if the body has decomposed, making all other examinations useless, but their absence does not mean that the body did not die from drowning.

The diatom test is plagued with difficulties and is not easy to carry out satisfactorily, for claims have been readily made, that diatoms can be discovered in non-drowned bodies, tap water, dust and even in the air!

Biochemical tests have been carried out on very fresh drowned bodies and by animal experimentation. The evidence seems to be that if a person drowns in salt water the osmotic concentration in the blood is greatly disturbed by the influx of the numerous elements and chemicals in the sea, thereby making the blood 'thick' or hypertonic. Death is considered to be much slower than in fresh water following marked chemical imbalances.

On the other hand, if a person drowns in fresh water, the 'pure' water dilutes the circulating blood and the electrolyte concentrations in the blood are reduced. Haemolysis rapidly takes place thereby reducing the oxygen carrying capacity of the blood. Death is achieved in a relatively short time from anoxia in addition to the asphyxial component caused by water in the air passages and the reflex closure of the larynx.

Death by immersion

On entry into the water, death may occur very rapidly,

almost instantaneously, so that it is proper for one to say that death was due to a reflex cardiac arrest. The back of the nose, the pharynx, larynx, in particular the vocal cords and the upper part of the trachea are very sensitive to unexpected stimuli. They are adequately supplied by branches of the vagus nerve. Should such an area receive a sudden unexpected stimulus, such as the impact of cold water, then the resultant 'shock' is reflected along the whole pathway of the vagus nerve(s) resulting in vagal over-stimulation of its many branches, including that to the heart. The dramatic effect is the sudden death of the victim.

Example A primary school class was having a swimming lesson at the local swimming baths. The young children were standing in a line on the edge of the bath, at the shallow end, and the teacher was standing in the water facing them. Two of the boys were slightly misbehaving with the result that one of them slipped off the edge and dropped feet first into the water, fairly close to the teacher. He slumped to the bottom of the pool and remained motionless. Despite immediate first aid measures by the teacher, he had died, without any struggle or signs of drowning. He had died from reflex cardiac arrest following immersion.

Other examples regularly encountered include alcoholics who fall into the canal, or river, people slipping off the decks of boats and people slipping under the water in their baths. At autopsy, there is nothing abnormal to be seen, certainly none of the pulmonary characteristics associated with drowning. The diagnosis is made from the circumstances.

Among other contributory factors to death by

drowning, are the presence of alcohol or other drugs in the body, the strong association of cold water and hypothermia, fear, inability to swim and the encumbrance of heavy or awkward clothing.

In summary, the examination and investigation of a body recovered from the water usually raises more questions than answers can be given and more research into deaths by immersion and drowning needs to be done urgently.

SUGGESTED FURTHER READING

Camps, F.E. (ed.) (1976), *Gradwohl's Legal Medicine* (3rd end), John Wright, Bristol.

Knight, B. (1985), *Pocket Guide to Forensic Medicine*. Heinemann Medical Books, London.

Knight, B. (1987), *Legal Aspects of Medical Practice* (4th edn), Churchill Livingstone, London.

Mant, A.K. (ed.) (1964), *Taylor's Principles and Practice of Medical Jurisprudence*. Churchill Livingstone, London.

Mason, J.K. (1983), *Forensic Medicine for Lawyers* (2nd edn), Butterworth, London.

Polsen, C., Gee, D. & Knight, B. (1985), *Essentials of Forensic Medicine* (4th edn), Pergamon Press, Oxford.

Simpson, C.K. & Knight, B. (1985), *Forensic Medicine* (9th edn), Arnold, London.

The list is clearly a personal one, and is by no means exhaustive.

INDEX

abdomen 90-91
  distension of 85
abdominal
  aorta 118
  enlargements 11
accidental cut-throats 158
adipocere 62
adrenal, haemorrhage 126
adulthood 29
age 25
air passages, haemorrhage in the 120
air weapons 254
alcohol 311
  abuse of 249
  intoxication 177, 185
  levels in vitreous humour 56
Allied War Crimes Commission 6
amperage 222
amylase 57
anaesthetic, general 213
anal intercourse 302
aneurysm 115, 176

    aortic 119
    berry 124
    dissecting 119
animal induced 67
anorexia nervosa 'the slimmer's disease' 227
anticipation of shock 221
anus 85-6
aorta, abdominal 118
aortic valve disease 117
artefacts, post mortem 51
arteries, vertebral 176
asphyxia
    environmental 202
    mechanical 182
    medically induced 204
    sexual 187
    toxic 195
    traumatic (crush) 197
assault
    indecent 287
    sexual 146
asthma 122
atheroma 114
atherosclerosis, coronary 117
attendant, mortuary 78
attitude, pugilistic 49, 241
autolysis 59
autopsy 72
    cremation 75
    forensic 74
    hospital 73
    private 76

baby, battered 280
bacterial activity 59

bacterial endocarditis 117
bags, brown paper 80
   polythene container 183
barrels, rifled or grooved 254
battered
   baby 280
   child 280
   child syndrome 280
   grannies 227
before entry
birth, inattention at 276
bite-marks 38
blast injuries 232
blast wave, effects of 233
blood pressure, raised 116
Bluebottle, Common 65
body
   obese 53
   resistance of the 223
   thin 54
bone defects 7
   hyoid 190, 191, 194
bones 17
   long 25
bronchopneumonia, haemorrhagic 122
bronchospasm 122
Brown House moth 63
brown paper bags 80
bruises, contusions 139
burns 10, 133
   flame and heat 238
   flash 215
   metallic 215

cadaveric spasm 51, 157

calf muscles 93
carbon dioxide 203
carbon monoxide 45, 247
    intoxication 199
    poisoning 45
carboxyhaemoglobin 201
cardiac deaths, reflex 127
cardiomyopathy 118
cartilage, thyroid 190, 191, 194
cartridge case 263
cases, civil 1
centres
    ossification 33
    vital 201
cerebral
    haemorrhage 123
    thrombus 124
certain direction 135
Certificate of Still-birth 109
certified midwife 110
charting of teeth 37
chemical thermometer 52
chemicals, corrosive 10
chest, surface of the 85
child, battered 280
childhood 32
cholinesterases 57
choking 185
chronic physical disease
Circle of Willis 124, 176
cirrhosis of liver 126
civil cases 1
clinician induced 69
closed circuit television 4
closed head injury 179

Clostridia 59
Clostridium welchii 62
clothing 5
cold water 310
Common
    Bluebottle 65
    Housefly 66
concussion 173
consent to the examination 290
contact
    mark 224
    wound 260
contents of pocket 5
contrecoup 178
contusions, bruises 139
cooling curve 52
cord
    spinal 93
    umbilical 192
coronary atherosclerosis 117
corrosive chemicals 10
cot death – Sudden Infant Death Syndrome 278
cough reflex 186
cremation autopsy 75
criminal act 306
(crush) traumatic asphyxia 197
cut-throat 154
    accidental 158
    suicidal 154
cyanide, hydrogen 248
cyanide
    intoxication 201
    poisoning 45

death by immersion 305, 306, 309-10

deceased 1
decomposition 13, 59
defects
   bone 7
   personal 7
   skin 7
definite pattern 135
dental records 38
dentures 38
depletion, oxygen 237
depressed fracture 170
desquamation 245
destruction, total body 232
development of foetus 29
diatoms 308-9
direct measurement 12
disease 221
   aortic valve 117
   chronic physical 306
   hypertensive heart 116
   industrial 205
   ischaemic heart 113
   rheumatic heart 117
dissecting aneurysm 119
dissection, medico-legal 72
distention of abdomen 85
domestic and industrial fires 199
dry heat 216
duodenal ulcer, gastric or 125
dura mater 173

earthing 223
electrical path 224
electrophoresis, immuno- 58
embolism, pulmonary 119

endocarditis, bacterial 117
enlargements, abdominal 11
entombment 227
environmental
   asphyxia 202
   temperature 55
enzyme determination, post mortem 57
epilepsy 125
epilepticus, status 125
epiphyses, fusion of 33
examination
   consent to the 290
   post mortem 72
   regional 88
   x-ray 86
exhaustion, heat 211
existence, separate 272
exits, access to 251
explosions 230
   industrial 231
exposure, hypothermia and 45
external genitalia 85-6
extradural
   haemorrhage 171
   heat haematoma 246
   space 173
extra-uterine pregnancy 126
eyelids 83
eyes 83

facial outlines 6
famine 228
fatty change to the liver 126
female pelvic organs 92
fingerprints 39

firearms, rifled 261
fires, domestic and industrial 199
flame and heat burns 238
'flash'
  burns 215
  marks 225
fluid, seminal 292
flying missiles, injuries from 233
foetus 25
  development of 29
forensic autopsy 74
Form
  A 105
  B 105
  C 106
  D 107
  E 108
  F 107
  G 107
  H – England, Wales & Scotland 108
  H – Northern Ireland 109
  I 109
formal identification 4
formalities of identifying 78
formation, gas 60
formulae, mathematical 13
fracture
  depressed 170
  heat 245
  simple 169
freezing, effects of 49
frenum 84
freshwater 309
froth 308
full term 272

full term or premature 272
fusion of epiphyses 33

gagging 184
gas formation 60
gastric or duodenal ulcer 125
general anaesthetic 213
genital organs, male 93
genitalia, external 85-6
Glaister Keen rods 299
'goose skin'
grannies, battered 227
Greenbottle 66
gums 64
gun-shot wounds 259

haematoma, extradural heat 246
haemorrhage
    adrenal 126
    cerebral 123
    extradural 171
    in the air passages 120
    intracerebral 178
    intracranial 124, 177
    petechial 189, 191, 195
    profuse 153
    subarachnoid 175
    subdural 174
haemorrhagic bronchopneumonia 122
hair 38
    to the laboratory 39
hands and arms, surfaces of 85
hanging 186
head, injuries to the 245
heart, silent rupture of 116

heat
  dry 216
  effects of excess 49
  exhaustion 211
  fractures 245
  hyperpyrexia 212
  moist 217
  stroke 54, 212
hide-and-die syndrome 210
homicidal cut-throat 157
homosexual offences 288
hormone levels, study of 57
hospital autopsy 73
Housefly, Common 66
hydrogen cyanide 248
hydrostatic test 274
hymenal injury 298
hyperinflated lungs 308
hyperpyrexia, malignant 213
hypertension, primary or essential 116
hypertensive heart disease 116
hyperthermia 211
hypostasis 46
  post mortem 143, 144
hypothermia 54, 202, 206, 207, 208, 209
  and exposure 45
hyoid bone 19, 191, 194

identification, formal 4
identifying, formalities of 78
immersion, sudden 305, 309-10
immuno-electrophoresis 58
impact, point of 135, 139
inattention at birth 276
incest 288

incisions
   primary 87
   surgical 153
indecent assault 287
industrial
   diseases 205
   explosions 231
infant, new born 32
infants 29
infarction, myocardial 114
infections 121
injuries
   blast 232
   due to the explosion itself 232
   from flying missiles 233
injuries to the head 245
   respiratory tract 244
injury
   closed head 179
   hymenal 298
   severe internal 138
internal combustion engines 200
intercourse
   anal 302
   with girl under 16 286
interval, lucid 174
intoxication
   alcohol 177, 185
   carbon monoxide 199
   cyanide 201
intracerebral haemorrhages 178
intracranial haemorrhage 124, 177

kick 150
knot, slip 189

larvae 67
Law of Evidence in Scotland 77
lewd and libidinous practices 288
ligature
   mark 188
   strangulation 190
lightening 214
limbs, lower 86
lines, suture 170
lipid substances 57
lips 84
liver
   cirrhosis of 126
   fatty change to the 126
lividity 43
livor mortis 42
long bones 25
lucid interval 174
lucidity 175

male genital organs 92-3
malignant hyperpyrexia 213
malnutrition 229
manual strangulation (throttling) 192
mark
   bite 38
   contact 224
   flash 225
   ligature 188
   spark 225
   tattoo 8
   tentative 155
   torture 157
mathematical formulae 13

measurement direct 12
mechanical asphyxia 182
medical referee 107
medically induced asphyxia 204
medico-legal dissection 72
membrane, subarachnoid 175
meningococcal septicaemia 126
mental state 306
metallic burns 215
midwife, certified 110
middle ear haemorrhages 308
moist heat 217
monoxide, carbon 45, 247
mortis, livor 42
mortuary 79
mortuary attendant 78
moth, Brown House 63
mugging 196
mummification 63
muscles, calf 93
myocardial infarction 114

nail scrapings or clippings 82
natural diseases scars 11
necropsy 72
neglect 226
new born, infant 32
non-ionizing solar radiation 213

obese body 53
objects, personal 3
offences, homosexual 288
ossification centres 33
outlines, facial 6
overcrowding 203

overlaying 183
oxygen depletion 237

parchmenting 138
particles, soot 245
path, electrical 224
patterns definite 135
pelvic organs, female 92
pelvis 18
perineum 85-6
personal
   defects 7
   objects 3
petechial haemorrhages 189, 191, 195
phenol 219
phosphatases 57
photographs 131
pistol, self loading or automatic 263
placenta praevia 126
pneumothorax 121
pocket, contents of 5
point of impact 135, 139
poisoning
   carbon monoxide 45, 247
   cyanide 45
polythene container bags 183
popping, skin 11
post mortem
   artefacts 51, 67
   enzyme determination 57
   examination(s) 72
   hypostasis 143, 144
   staining hypostasis 42
potassium level, vitreous humour 56
primary or essential hypertension 116

primary incisions 87
printed protocols 130
private autopsy 76
procedures, special 92
pregnancy, extra-uterine 126
premature, full term or 272
proteins, serum 58
protocols, printed 130
'pugilistic' attitude 49, 241
pulmonary embolism 119
purpura, senile 143

radiation 218
   non-ionizing solar 213
raised blood pressure 116
rape 286
reaction, vital 138, 244
records, dental 38
recovery 307
referee, medical 107
reflex
   cardiac arrest 310
   cardiac deaths 127
   cough 186
regional examinations 88
resistance of the body 223
respiratory tract injuries 244
restraint, sites of 146
revolver 262
rheumatic heart disease 117
rifled firearms 261
rifled or grooved barrels 254
rigidity 47
rings 5
'rule of nines' 241

ruptured aortic aneurysm 118

sacrum 22
salt water 309
samples, swab 81
scalp 83, 146, 168
scapulae 145
scars 9
    following violence 10
    natural diseases 11
    self injection 10
    surgical 10
self-loading or automatic pistol 263
seminal fluid 292
senile purpura 143
separate existence, still-birth or 272
septicaemia, meningococcal 126
serum proteins 58
severe internal injuries 138
sexual
    asphyxia 187
    assaults 146
shock, anticipation of 221
shotgun 255
    wound 259
silent rupture of heart 116
simple fracture 169
sites of restraint 146
skeleton 91
skin
    defects 7
    slip 60
'skin-popping' 11
skull 23, 169
slip knot 189

smoke 238
smooth-barrelled weapons 254
soot particles 245
space, extradural 173
spark mark 225
spasm, cadaveric 51, 157
special procedures 91
spermatozoa 292
spinal cord 93
spots, Tardieu's 46
sprung suture 170
stab wound 160, 162
staining hypostasis, post mortem 42
starvation 226
stature 12
status epilepticus 125
statutory definition of either a wound or injury 129
sternum 23
still-birth or separate existence 272
    certificate of 109
stimulation, vagal 186, 192
strangulation
    ligature 190
    (throttling) manual 192
stroke 179
    heat 54, 212
study of hormone levels 57
stump, umbilical 275
subarachnoid
    haemorrhage 175
    membrane 175
subdural haemorrhage 174
substances, lipid 57
sudden immersion 305, 309-10
Sudden Infant Death Syndrome (cot death) 183, 278

suffocation 182
suicidal cut-throat wound 154
surgical
    incision 153
    scars 10
suspension 186
suture
    lines 170
    sprung 187
swab
    samples 81
    vaginal 297

Tardieu's spots 46
tattoo marks 8
teeth 84
    charting of 37
television, closed circuit 4
temperature, environmental 55
tentative marks 155
thermometer, chemical 52
thin body 54
thorax 89-90
thrombo-phlebitis 119
thrombus, cerebral 124
thyroid cartilage 190, 191, 194
torture marks 157
total body destruction 232
toxic asphyxia 195
transaminases 57
traumatic (crush) asphyxia 197

ulcer, gastric or duodenal 125
umbilical
    cord 192

stump 275

vagal stimulation 186, 192
vaginal swabs 297
ventilation, inadequate 200
vertebral arteries 176
violence, scars following 10
virginity 291
vital
    centres 201
    reaction 138, 244
vitreous humour 58
    alcohol levels 56
    potassium level 56
voltage 221

'washerwoman's hands'
weapons
    air 254
    rifled 261
    smooth-barrelled 254
Willis, Circle of 124, 176
wound
    contact 260
    gun-shot 259
    homicidal cut-throat 157
    or injury, statutory definition of either 129
    shotgun 255
    stab 160, 162
    suicidal cut-throat 154

x-ray examination 86